EMDR Therapy and EMERGENCY RESPONSE

Marilyn Luber, PhD, is a licensed clinical psychologist in general private practice in Center City, Philadelphia, Pennsylvania. She was trained in eye movement desensitization and reprocessing (EMDR) in 1992 by Dr. Francine Shapiro, and now assists in EMDR Institute trainings as a facilitator and logistics coordinator. She has coordinated trainings in EMDR-related fields in the greater Philadelphia area since 1997. She teaches Facilitator and Supervisory trainings and other EMDR-related subjects both nationally and internationally, and was on the EMDR Task Force for Dissociative Disorders. She was on the founding board of directors of the EMDR International Association (EMDRIA) and served as the chair of the International Committee until June 1999. Currently, she is a facilitator in the EMDR Global Alliance, a group consisting of the leaders of all the EMDR associations who are working to support standards in EMDR worldwide. In 1997, Dr. Luber was given a Humanitarian Services Award by the EMDR Humanitarian Association, and later, in 2003, she was presented with the EMDR International Association's award for "outstanding contribution and service to EMDRIA." In 2005, she was awarded the Francine Shapiro Award for "outstanding contribution and service to EMDR." In 2009, she edited *Eye Movement Desensitization and Reprocessing (EMDR) Scripted Protocols: Basics and Special Situations* and *Eye Movement Desensitization and Reprocessing (EMDR) Scripted Protocols: Special Populations,* published by Springer Publishing Company. Several years later, in 2012, she edited Springer's first CD-ROM books, *Eye Movement Desensitization and Reprocessing (EMDR) Scripted Protocols With Summary Sheets CD-ROM Version: Basics and Special Situations* and *Eye Movement Desensitization and Reprocessing (EMDR) Scripted Protocols With Summary Sheets CD-ROM Version: Special Populations*. In 2001, through EMDR-HAP (Humanitarian Assistance Programs), she published *Handbook for EMDR Clients* and it has been translated into eight languages. She has written the "Around the World" and "In the Spotlight" articles for the EMDRIA Newsletter four times a year since 1997. She has worked as a primary consultant for the FBI field division in Philadelphia. Dr. Luber has a general psychology practice, working with adolescents, adults, and couples, especially with complex post-traumatic stress disorder (C-PTSD), trauma and related issues, and dissociative disorders. She runs consultation groups for EMDR practitioners.

EMDR Therapy and EMERGENCY RESPONSE

Edited by

Marilyn Luber, PhD

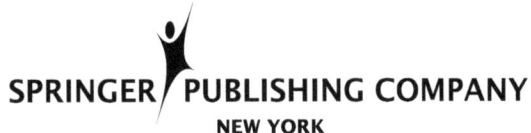

SPRINGER PUBLISHING COMPANY
NEW YORK

Copyright © 2015 Springer Publishing Company, LLC

All rights reserved.

No part of this publication may be reproduced, stored in a retrieval system, or transmitted in any form or by any means, electronic, mechanical, photocopying, recording, or otherwise, without the prior permission of Springer Publishing Company, LLC, or authorization through payment of the appropriate fees to the Copyright Clearance Center, Inc., 222 Rosewood Drive, Danvers, MA 01923, 978-750-8400, fax 978-646-8600, info@copyright.com or on the Web at www.copyright.com.

Springer Publishing Company, LLC
11 West 42nd Street
New York, NY 10036
www.springerpub.com

Acquisitions Editor: Sheri W. Sussman
Composition: S4Carlisle

ISBN: 978-0-8261-3337-3
e-book ISBN: 978-0-8261-3223-9

Content herein is excerpted from *Implementing EMDR Early Mental Health Interventions for Man-Made and Natural Disasters: Models, Scripted Protocols, and Summary Sheets*, edited by Marilyn Luber. © Springer Publishing Company, LLC. The Foreword, Preface, Acknowledgments, and section introductions have been included herein in their entirety.

The author and the publisher of this Work have made every effort to use sources believed to be reliable to provide information that is accurate and compatible with the standards generally accepted at the time of publication. The author and publisher shall not be liable for any special, consequential, or exemplary damages resulting, in whole or in part, from the readers' use of, or reliance on, the information contained in this book. The publisher has no responsibility for the persistence or accuracy of URLs for external or third-party Internet websites referred to in this publication and does not guarantee that any content on such websites is, or will remain, accurate or appropriate.

Implementing EMDR early mental health interventions for man-made and natural disasters : models, scripted protocols, and summary sheets/edited by Marilyn Luber.
    p. ; cm.
  Implementing eye movement desensitization reprocessing early mental health interventions for man-made and natural disasters
  Includes bibliographical references and index.
  ISBN-13: 978-0-8261-9921-8
  ISBN-10: 0-8261-9921-6
  ISBN-13: 978-0-8261-3223-9 (e-book)
  ISBN-13: 978-0-8261-2957-4 (CD-ROM)
    I. Luber, Marilyn, editor of compilation. II. Title: Implementing eye movement desensitization reprocessing early mental health interventions for man-made and natural disasters.
  [DNLM: 1. Stress Disorders, Traumatic—therapy. 2. Cross-Cultural Comparison. 3. Disasters. 4. Eye Movement Desensitization Reprocessing. WM 172.5]
  RC552.T7
  616.85'21—dc23
                      2013021409

Special discounts on bulk quantities of our books are available to corporations, professional associations, pharmaceutical companies, health care organizations, and other qualifying groups.

If you are interested in a custom book, including chapters from more than one of our titles, we can provide that service as well.

For details, please contact:
Special Sales Department, Springer Publishing Company, LLC
11 West 42nd Street, 15th Floor, New York, NY 10036-8002
Phone: 877-687-7476 or 212-431-4370; Fax: 212-941-7842
E-mail: sales@springerpub.com

Printed in the United States of America.

To my mother, who has been going through her own recent trauma
with the spirit and true determination
that she has always displayed throughout her life:
a role model for us all.

Epigraph

We are all responsible for the world we live in. Worldwide, clinicians are forging bonds that transcend countries and ideologies. Bonds that can help heal the trauma and pain that lead to ongoing violence and suffering. To make a difference that effects generations to come—don't leave it to anyone else. We all have to take a part in it.

—Francine Shapiro

Contents

Contributors xi

Foreword xv
Robert Gelbach

Preface xvii

Acknowledgments xxxi

PART I
EMDR On-Site or Hospital Response

Chapter 1 Emergency Response Procedure (ERP) 3
Gary Quinn

Summary Sheet: Emergency Response Procedure (ERP) 13
Marilyn Luber

Chapter 2 EMDR Emergency Room and Wards Protocol (EMDR-ER©) 17
Judith S. B. Guedalia and Frances R. Yoeli

Summary Sheet: EMDR Emergency Room and Wards Protocol (EMDR-ER©) 27
Marilyn Luber

PART II
EMDR Early Intervention Procedures for Individuals

Chapter 3 The Recent Traumatic Episode Protocol (R-TEP):
An Integrative Protocol for Early EMDR Intervention (EEI) 35
Elan Shapiro and Brurit Laub

Summary Sheet: The Recent Traumatic Episode Protocol (R-TEP):
An Integrative Protocol for Early EMDR Intervention (EEI) 51
Marilyn Luber

Chapter 4 The EMDR Protocol for Recent Critical Incidents (EMDR-PRECI) 59
Ignacio Jarero and Lucina Artigas

Summary Sheet: The EMDR Protocol for Recent
Critical Incidents (EMDR–PRECI) 71
Marilyn Luber

PART III
EMDR Early Intervention for Groups

Chapter 5 **The EMDR Integrative Group Treatment Protocol (IGTP) for Children** 79
Lucina Artigas, Ignacio Jarero, Nicté Alcalá, and Teresa López Cano

Summary Sheet for Each Participant: The EMDR Integrative Group Treatment Protocol (IGTP) for Children 87
Marilyn Luber

Summary Sheet for Clinicians: The EMDR Integrative Group Treatment Protocol (IGTP) for Children 91
Marilyn Luber

Chapter 6 **The EMDR Integrative Group Treatment Protocol (IGTP) for Adults** 95
Ignacio Jarero and Lucina Artigas

Summary Sheet for Each Participant: The EMDR Integrative Group Treatment Protocol (IGTP) for Adults 103
Marilyn Luber

Summary Sheet for Clinicians: The EMDR Integrative Group Treatment Protocol (IGTP) for Adults 105
Marilyn Luber

Appendix A: Worksheets 109

Appendix B: EMDR Worldwide Associations and Other Resources 128

References and Bibliography 135

Contributors

Nicté Alcalá, MA, has been working with survivors of traumatic events during her professional life. The clients with whom she has been working the most are those who have suffered from complex interpersonal trauma, rape, assault, robbery, kidnapping, and natural or human-provoked disasters. She has been involved in humanitarian projects in Latin America since 1998. Her private practice is in Mexico City.

Lucina Artigas, MA, MT, is a trainer of trainers, and an EMDRIA and EMDR-Ibero-America–approved consultant. She is cofounder and executive director of EMDR-Mexico, AMAMECRISIS, and International Center of Psychotraumatology. In 2000, she received the EMDRIA Creative Innovation Award for the Butterfly Hug, and, in 2007, she received the EMDR-Ibero-America Francine Shapiro Award. She is a trainer for the International Critical Incident Stress Foundation and Green Cross Academy of Traumatology. She is coauthor of the EMDR Integrative Group Treatment Protocol that has been applied successfully with disaster survivors worldwide. She has presented workshops and has published articles on EMDR, Crisis Intervention, and Compassion Fatigue. Since 1997, she has been involved in humanitarian projects in Latin America and Europe.

Teresa López Cano, MA, has worked with survivors of traumatic events throughout her professional career. She treats clients who have suffered from complex interpersonal trauma, rape, assault, robbery, kidnapping, and natural or human-provoked disasters. Since 1998, she has been actively involved in humanitarian projects in Latin America. Her private practice is in Mexico City.

Judith S. B. Guedalia, PhD, is a senior medical psychologist and a member of the ER (emergency room) trauma staff in times of mass community events (MCE, or ARAN, the Hebrew acronym). She is Director of Shaare Zedek Medical Center's Neuropsychology Unit; among the many situations the Neuropsychology Unit has treated are emotional trauma, anxiety, depression, parenting and family issues, stress, issues concerning children of divorce, self-esteem issues, patient adjustment to neurological or cognitive problems, adjustment to chronic illness, family adjustment to and coping with a member's illness, and adjustment to developmental disabilities. Dr. Guedalia is an EMDR therapist and is in the process of completing the requirements to be a supervisor of other EMDR therapists. Dr. Guedalia is the founder and co-chair of Nefesh Israel, the Israeli branch of the NEFESH International Organization, the Networking Association for Orthodox Mental Health Professionals. She has published in peer-reviewed journals in neuropsychology, Judaism, and mental health. She is also a regular columnist for ***The Jewish Press,*** America's largest independent Jewish weekly. She was born in New York City, and has studied and worked in New York, New York; London, England; Holyoke, Massachusetts; Los Angeles, California; and Jerusalem, Israel (since 1980).

Ignacio Jarero, PhD, EdD, MT, is a trainer of trainers, EMDRIA and EMDR-Ibero-America cofounder, and approved consultant. He is cofounder and president of EMDR-Mexico, AMAMECRISIS, and International Center of Psychotraumatology. In 2007, he received the EMDR-Ibero-America Francine Shapiro Award and, in 2008, the Argentinian Society of Psychotrauma (ISTSS Affiliate) awarded him the Psychotrauma Trajectory Award. He is a trainer for the International Critical Incident Stress Foundation and Green Cross Academy of Traumatology. Dr. Jarero is coauthor of the EMDR Integrative Group Treatment Protocol that has been applied successfully with disaster survivors worldwide. He has presented workshops and has published articles on EMDR, crisis intervention, and compassion fatigue. Since 1997, he has been involved in humanitarian projects in Latin America and Europe.

Brurit Laub, PhD, is a senior clinical psychologist, with over 30 years of experience working in community mental health in Israel. She was also a teacher and supervisor at the Machon Magid School of Psychotherapy at Hebrew University in Jerusalem and at different marriage and family counseling centers. She is an accredited hypnotherapist, and a supervisor in psychotherapy and family therapy. She presents workshops concerning models developed independently and, together with colleagues, on narrative therapy, script changing therapy, coping with monsters, dialectical cotherapy, and a transgenerational tool. Dr. Laub works with subpersonalities nationally and internationally. She has published 15 articles on the above topics in international and Israeli journals. In 1994, she coauthored, with S. Hoffman and S. Gafni, "Co-Therapy With Individuals, Families." In 2006, she collaborated again with S. Hoffman on "Innovative Interventions in Psychotherapy." In 1998, she became an EMDR facilitator and she is an EMDR-Europe–accredited consultant. Dr. Laub has been involved with HAP trainings in Turkey and Sri Lanka. She developed a Resource Connection Envelope (RCE) for the Standard EMDR Protocol and presented it in workshops and for EMDR conferences in Tel-Aviv, London, Vancouver, Denver, Istanbul, and Norway. With Esti Bar-Sade, she developed the Imma EMDR Group Protocol, which is an adaptation of Artigas, Jarero, Alcalá, and López's IGTP. Together with Elan Shapiro, she presented their Recent Traumatic Episode Protocol (R-TEP) in Israel, Europe, and the United States. She coauthored two publications about the R-TEP protocol in the ***Journal of EMDR Practice and Research*** with Elan Shapiro and Nomi Weiner. She lives in Rehovot and is in private practice.

Gary Quinn, MD, is a psychiatrist and director of The Jerusalem EMDR Institute. He specializes in crisis intervention, the treatment of anxiety and depressive disorders, and the treatment of post-traumatic stress disorder following military trauma, terrorist attacks, and motor vehicle accidents. He is the cofounder, former co-chairman, and current vice chairman of EMDR-Israel. He has conducted numerous trainings in Israel and runs supervision groups. He is the trainer of trainers in Asia for the EMDR Institute Inc. and is a senior trainer in Asia and the United States. He participated as a trainer for HAP (Humanitarian Assistance Programs) in Turkey following the earthquake of 1999, in Thailand after the tsunami in 2004, and in Romania and Cambodia. He has volunteered in medical hospitals after terrorist attacks and treated patients with ASD and PTSD in bomb shelters using EMDR, EMD, and the group disaster protocol. He developed the Emergency Response Protocol (ERP) to treat victims of trauma with EMDR within hours of the incident, when patients are suffering from speechless terror with multiple rapid flashbacks. Dr. Quinn has presented this work at a conference in trauma (United Kingdom and Ireland), at the EMDR Society (Glasgow, Scotland), to the World Psychiatric Association Regional (Seoul, South Korea), and at the EMDR European Conferences (Paris, London, Amsterdam, and Vienna). He was invited to Singapore as a PTSD expert to address the psychiatric, psychological, and medical staff as well as policy makers from the Department of Mental Health. He was the keynote speaker at the Singapore International Conference on treatment of acute stress disorder. He served as a consultant in the Ohio State University Stress, Trauma and Resilience (STAR) Program and has presented at Grand Rounds on "EMDR, PTSD, and Medical Systems Trauma" at Ohio State University Department of Psychiatry.

Elan Shapiro, MA, is a psychologist in private practice in Israel with over 30 years of experience. He worked as a senior consulting psychologist in a Community Psychological Service in Upper Nazareth. Originally specializing in Adlerian psychology, he came to EMDR in 1989 after attending one of the first trainings ever given. In 1994, after additional training in the United States and Europe, he became an EMDR facilitator. He was among the founding members of EMDR-Europe, EMDR-Israel, and a charter member of EMDRIA. He is an EMDR-Europe–accredited consultant and was secretary of EMDR-Europe for 8 years. He is currently co–vice president of EMDR Israel. He has been involved with HAP trainings in Turkey, Sri Lanka, and Thailand. He and Brurit Laub have presented their Recent Traumatic Episode Protocol (R-TEP) training workshop to over a thousand EMDR practitioners in Israel, Europe, and the United States. They also presented R-TEP for the EMDR-Europe Consultants day at the EMDR-Europe Annual Conference in London (2008); preconference workshops at EMDRIA's annual conferences in Atlanta (2009) and Minneapolis (2010), as well as for the EMDR Institute in San Diego and Denver in 2012. He has authored and coauthored a number of articles including an invited article on Early EMDR Intervention for the special 20-year anniversary issue of the *Journal of EMDR Practice and Research* in 2009.

Frances R. Yoeli, MSc, MFT, CAC, LISW, is a certified traumatologist, EMDR-HAP facilitator, and consultant for the Life Energy Center in Israel. Her clinical experience has spanned three continents and four decades. She works with PTSD from abuse, wars, mass disasters, terrorism, critical incidents, and traumatic events. Other specialties include anxiety, eating disorders, addictions, new religious movement issues, cults, ritual abuse with trauma victims, couples, families, and clients presenting with depressions, loss, grief, and the full range of psychosomatic and dissociative disorders. She headed the Emergency Mental Health Team in the Emek Bet-Shean Valley for many years. As a HAP facilitator and consultant, she faced several Asian challenges in humanitarian field work, and facilitated EMDR trainings in the region. For 6 years, she worked as coordinator for HAP events in Israel. Dr. Yoeli has given numerous presentations in professional conferences on EMDR, dissociation, cult and ritual abuse, and terrorism worldwide. With her colleague Tessa Prattos from Greece, she completed the book chapter "Terrorism Is the Ritual Abuse of the Twenty-First Century" in the book *Ritual Abuse in the 21st Century* (2008), edited by Randy Noblitt and Pamala Perskin Noblitt. They are refining their "Multi-Tiered Trans-Generational Genogram," which is part of their EMDR-AIR Protocol, cooperating with the International Trauma Center in Athens, Greece, and with the Functional Medical Center in Minneapolis, Minnesota, on its clinical application. She is currently researching her work from a Conversation Analysis perspective, collaborating with Dr. Alan Zemel, PhD, University of Albany, and with psychologist Tessa Prattos, MA, in Athens, Greece.

Foreword

Foreword taken from *Implementing EMDR Early Mental Health Interventions for Man-Made and Natural Disasters: Models, Scripted Protocols, and Summary Sheets*, edited by Marilyn Luber. © Springer Publishing Company, LLC.

Human beings are born into the care and company of others. From our first breath, our lives are a progressive encounter and mastery of enviroming stresses, mediated to an overwhelming degree by the web of social relationships and cultural meanings that sustain us throughout our lives. Sometimes, our individual capacity to manage excessive stress derails us and we may need assistance to reestablish a healthy coping capability. The evolution of mental health resources in developed countries has expanded the availability and efficacy of such assistance for individuals overcome by personal traumatic stress in normal times.

But disaster is not "normal"; in fact it is a severe disruption of the normal context in which we can find our bearings and rely on familiar systems of support. Disaster brings very high levels of traumatic stress at the same time that it undermines the usual coping resources and systems of care that may mitigate trauma or support healing.

The authors collected in this volume have been creative participants in the first generation of therapists who employed EMDR as a clinical treatment for posttraumatic stress disorder and related conditions. They know firsthand what research has confirmed—that EMDR is an effective and efficacious treatment for trauma in both children and adults, across all cultures and groups where it has been employed. It was only natural that they would want to apply this therapy to the massive trauma issues arising in modern day disasters, whether these arise from natural events (earthquake, tsunami, hurricane) or man-made disasters (warfare, flight from persecution, or famine).

However, although much psychotherapy has advanced in the past century in some parts of the world, it remains substantially underdeveloped where most of the world's people live. Moreover, even in places where psychotherapy is well-established it is not widely available at all socioeconomic levels. And most important, it is not widely understood by those who coordinate disaster response nationally or internationally that psychotherapy has a valuable role in early disaster intervention.

Clinician volunteers from the EMDR Humanitarian Assistance Program (HAP) and sister organizations have not been discouraged by these circumstances. As the following chapters recount, they have rolled up their sleeves and entered into the scene of disaster determined to find out how principles of EMDR can be best utilized to reduce trauma and increase the coping capacity of disaster survivors so that the goals of recovery and adaptation can be more fully and rapidly attained.

I had the privilege of meeting and working with many of the authors collected here while I served as Executive Director of HAP. They accomplished much by their direct service to survivors and by their teaching of useful skills to local caregivers. But they also learned much about the capacity of other cultures to support the coping efforts of their members, about the need for mental health response to blend collaboratively into the overall efforts of disaster responders to also address medical, nutritional, shelter, security, economic, and other needs. They learned the importance of adapting the mental health response to the particular phase of disaster recovery, and to the need for special attention to the first responders and local human service workers confronting vicarious traumatization.

Surely one of the most universal lessons learned was that populations and public officials everywhere were rarely equipped in advance to grapple with the emergent mental health issues that arise out of a community-wide disaster. From this recognition has come a growing effort to develop in all countries a more widespread understanding of traumatic stress and its treatment. Especially because disasters tend to occur in those countries and populations that are least resilient, the efforts to build up public understanding of trauma and caregiver skills for stress reduction **before disaster strikes** seem most likely to mitigate the psychological toll of future disasters. That is why HAP has been particularly interested in developing Trauma Recovery Networks in all countries where HAP works.

In this latest insightful volume gathered and edited by Marilyn Luber, the authors have combined the lessons learned with personal accounts of how they proceeded. There is still much to be done to integrate mental health care effectively into disaster response worldwide, but this volume will help to point the way to best practices.

Robert Gelbach, PhD
Past Executive Director at EMDR Humanitarian Assistance Programs

Preface

Preface taken from *Implementing EMDR Early Mental Health Interventions for Man-Made and Natural Disasters: Models, Scripted Protocols, and Summary Sheets*, edited by Marilyn Luber. © Springer Publishing Company, LLC.

All of us familiar with EMDR have heard about Francine Shapiro's 1987 walk in the park and how she observed her own disturbing thoughts disappear. On reflection, she realized that her eye movements seemed to be resulting in a decrease of her once distressing thoughts. She was surprised and intrigued and tried it again with other thoughts. It worked again. She decided to try it with friends, and when it worked again, she tried it with clients. She took this eye movement phenomenon and crafted a protocol based on the following elements:

- Incident: "Describe the memory from which you wish relief in terms of who was involved and what had happened."
- Picture: "Isolate a single picture that represents the entire memory (preferably the most traumatic point of the incident) and indicate who and what is in the picture."
- Negative cognition (NC): "What words about yourself or the incident best go with the picture?"
- SUD scale: "Imagine the traumatic scene and the words of the belief statement ___ (state the negative cognition) and assign a SUDs (subjective units of disturbance scale) where 0 = (neutral or calm) to 10 = (the worst you can think of), how does it feel?"
- Positive cognition (PC): "How would you like to feel instead?"
- Validity of cognition (VoC) for PC: On a 1 to 7 scale where 1 feels completely false and 7 feels completely true, how true does the new statement feel to you?" (Shapiro, 1989)

She called it Eye Movement Desensitization (EMD). Over time, as she observed the processing of many traumatic incidents by many clients, she believed that the results went beyond a desensitization effect and actually reprocessed and changed clients' perceptions of their traumas; she added an "R" for "Reprocessing" and renamed EMD to EMDR (Shapiro, 1991).

In 1989, the San Francisco Bay Area earthquake not only disrupted this community, it changed the way Francine viewed trauma that had recently/just occurred. As more and more clients came to her office to process their experiences of the quake, she noticed that something was different when she used her normal protocol for EMDR: It was not generalizing. Instead of targeting the memory and having the process link to the other associations related to the traumatic memory network, she had to be more actively engaged in helping clients target the next part of their earthquake experience. It was as if the parts were not yet integrated into a whole. She realized that the memories her clients were telling her had not yet consolidated and that she needed to figure out how to help them link into the memory networks associated with the event. The premise of EMDR is the Adaptive Information Processing Model (AIP; for more in-depth descriptions, see Shapiro, 1995, 2001, 2006; Shapiro, Kaslow, & Maxfield, 2007); this means that everyone has an inborn predisposition to move toward health and the internal ability to accomplish it. When this movement is obstructed (and not related to a lack of information or organic issues), it is probable that the experiences become dysfunctionally stored and unable to connect with other adaptive information. As a result, clients may have maladaptive images, perceptual distortions, emotions, and sensations that are "stuck" in trauma time, unable to process. That is, adaptive information is unable to link into the memory networks holding the dysfunctionally stored information. The goal becomes to enable the more adaptive information held in other neural networks to link into these dysfunctionally stored memories and facilitate normal memory processing.

In response to her clients' needs, she created the Protocol for Recent Traumatic Events (Shapiro, 1995; 2001). The protocol she crafted addressed how to reprocess the elements of an unconsolidated memory with little/no linkages. She started by obtaining a "narrative history" of the event. She wisely took each of the separate aspects of the memory her clients reported and treated each one of them as a separate target with the EMDR Standard procedure up to the installation of the positive cognition (PC). She thoughtfully decided to not go beyond that because clients would then have to pay attention to body sensations that would continue to be there, she reasoned, because the whole memory had yet to be completed. If there was a most disturbing element of the memory, she started there; if not, she followed clients' chronologies of the event. After the first part of the memory was completed, she did the others in chronological order.

To check the work, she asked clients to visualize the entire sequence of the event with their eyes closed as she figured they would be better able to concentrate on their experiences and associate to it. If they did notice that there was some residual distress, she asked them to stop and then she used the EMDR Procedure including the NC and PC. She had clients continue this process and repeat it—if needed—until the whole event could be experienced with no emotional, cognitive, or somatic change. By asking clients next to open their eyes and think of the whole event from start to finish, she could observe if they could also keep one foot in the present and one in the not-so-distant past. Then, she installed the PC. After this was done, she was ready to check and see if clients had any residual distress in their bodies that needed processing, so she had them do the body scan. When all of the different elements of the event were completed and the body scan was clear, she asked for any present stimuli such as triggers that resulted in a startle response, nightmares, or other reminders of the event that were still disturbing and she processed each trigger with her clients. Although she did not write about the future template in this section of her book, she discusses the 3-Pronged Protocol throughout it and so it is assumed that she includes this as well. Out of the devastating San Francisco Bay Area earthquake of 1989 came a new treatment for recent trauma.

Over the years, recognition of EMDR as a treatment has grown. In fact the following organizations are incorporating EMDR into their treatment guidelines: Clinical Division of the American Psychological Association (Chambless et al., 1998); United Kingdom Department of Health (2001); National Council for Mental Health (Israel) (Bleich, Kotler, Kutz, & Shalev, 2002); Clinical Resource Efficiency Support Team of the Northern Ireland Department of Health, Social Services and Public Safety, Belfast (CREST, 2003); Dutch National Steering Committee Guidelines Mental Health Care (2003); Stockholm: Medical Program Committee/Stockholm City Council, Sweden (Sjöblom et al., 2003); American Psychiatric Association (2004); Department of Veterans Affairs & Department of Defense (2004); French National Institute of Health and Medical Research (INSERM, 2004); Therapy Advisor (2004–2007); National Collaborating Center for Mental Health (2005); Australian Centre for Posttraumatic Mental Health (2007); Practice Guidelines of the International Society for Traumatic Stress Studies (Foa, 2009); California Evidence-Based Clearinghouse for Child Welfare (2010), and the Substance Abuse and Mental Health Services Administration (SAMHSA) National Registry of Evidence-Based Programs and Practices (SAMHSA, 2011) (retrieved from the EMDR Institute website [www.emdr.com] and Schubert & Lee [2009]). Only two of these guidelines include specific references to the use of EMDR with clients diagnosed with acute stress disorder (APA, 2004; Australian Centre for Posttraumatic Mental Health, 2007). The other guidelines designate EMDR as an evidence-based treatment for PTSD; however, it seems that all of the guidelines are referring to EMDR related to chronic PTSD (after 3 months).

Kutz, Resnick, and Dekel (2008) point out that information on "the biology and psychology of acute stress syndromes is relatively sparse," and they go on to suggest, based on their clinical experience with terror and accident victims, that the current idea of time-related definitions of acute, posttraumatic stress might need to be modified and gave the following example: "the border (4 weeks) between ASD and acute PTSD seems utterly arbitrary, and both ASD and acute PTSD seem to form a continuous acute stress (AS) syndrome." In a similar vein, Mark Russell, Tammera Cooke, and Susan Rogers in their chapter, "EMDR and Effective Management of Acute Stress Injuries: Early Mental Health Intervention From a Military Perspective" (Chapter 20) ask a similar question, "What is the difference between 3 weeks and 6 days (acute stress disorder) and 4 weeks and a day (PTSD)?" They note that after 4 weeks, the ASD diagnosis automatically converts to PTSD and EMDR is one of the few "A-level" trauma-targeted psychotherapies for PTSD. Also, they cite clinical case studies reported by Russell (2006) and Wesson and Gould (2009) showing that EMDR treatment is successful when treating combat-related ASR and ASD for those on active duty in the military. They believe that this distinction is arbitrary and empirically unsupported.

Elan Shapiro (2012, p. 244), in his article looking at the field of early psychological intervention (EPI) after trauma and the place of EMDR, reports, "the state of current evidence about early response to trauma and subsequent disorders reveals a complex picture. Bryant, Creamer, O'Donnell, Silove, and McFarlane (2011), summarizing the findings of an ambitious study which investigated the extent to which ASD at 1 month predicts posttraumatic psychiatric disorders at 12 months after trauma, in a large sample from five Australian hospitals concluded that the ASD diagnosis has limited utility in identifying recent trauma-exposed individuals who are at high risk for PTSD . . . however . . . most people diagnosed with ASD will suffer some psychiatric disorder a year later. . . . In contrast the overall utility of the diagnosis as an early screening strategy . . . is very limited because the majority of people who develop a disorder will not initially display full or subsyndromal ASD" (Bryant et al., 2011, p. 5).

Shapiro (2012, p. 244) discusses practical and ethical questions concerning the importance of treatment of ASD since so many go on to develop PTSD or other psychiatric disorders (Bryant, Friedman, Spiegel, Ursano, & Strain, 2010; Roberts, Kitchiner, Kenardy, & Bisson, 2009) and the fact that PTSD is only one of several disorders that can result from trauma may mean that we could be overlooking an important group who go on to develop these disorders. Shapiro goes on to report (2012, p. 244), "The possibility of delayed-onset PTSD should also be remembered, as it was found to occur in up to 68% of cases, depending on definitions (Andrews, Brewin, Philpott, & Stewart, 2007)." Other concerns, also in Shapiro's article (2012, p. 242), are mentioned by Vanitallie (2002), such as "the dysregulation of the metabolic system, stemming from chronic stress, and attempts to accommodate it (allostatic load) contributes to the development of a variety of illnesses, as well as certain disorders of immune function" or McFarlane (2010a, 2010b) who states, "The association with cardiovascular risk factors and inflammatory markers indicates that exposure to traumatic stress leads to a general disruption of an individual's underlying homeostasis" (2010b, p. 5). The high cost to individuals and to society is evident.

Although there are a number of PTSD studies concerning the efficacy of EMDR, there are very few reports on the effect of EMDR on AS; undoubtedly, more research would be helpful in more clearly defining these diagnoses and the best interventions for them. The Cochrane review of psychological interventions looked at psychological interventions within the first 3 months after a traumatic event, and was unable to recommend any early psychological intervention for general immediate use after a critical incident (Roberts, Kitchiner, Kenardy, & Bisson, 2008, 2009). However, EMDR-based protocols are being used with increasing frequency in individual or group formats to address the traumatic symptoms subsequent to man-made and natural disasters and from the reports and the research that is beginning to be published, survivors' traumatic symptoms are decreasing.

In this text, there are several different protocols used to address AS. Francine's original EMD Protocol was brought back into circulation in the *Military and Post-Disaster Response Manual* (Shapiro, 2004) for emergency situations such as in frontline military operations. In EMD, the client is returned to the target frequently, the SUD level is checked, and the focus is on the target without moving down the associative tracks to other events/situaions. This is a highly structured intervention meant to keep the client focused in emergency situations. Emergency room treatments have also been utilized as in Gary Quinn's Emergency Response Procedure (ERP) for stabilization (see Chapter 1) and Judith Guedalia and Frances Yoeli's EMDR Emergency Room and Wards Protocol (EMDR-ER©) (see Chapter 2) to help get patients who had been traumatized functioning again and able to leave the ER. Kutz, Resnick, and Dekel (2008) used a "modified, abridged, single session" EMDR protocol for AS syndromes using mainly the BLS element of the Standard EMDR Protocol without the cognitive processing elements while focusing on the most distressing sensory, bodily experience, or cognitive preoccupation related to the traumatic incident and rated with the SUDs. Sets are continued until there is a decrease in distress. Their results showed that with this intervention 50% had complete relief and 27% experienced substantial relief of their acutely stressed patients and concluded that this brief variation can be useful for victims of large scale disaster as well as trauma victims in hospitals and outpatient situations. Russell (see Chapter 20) has used EMD; he targets only a single memory with the image, NC, emotions, SUDs, and location of body sensation with BLS to assist with crisis intervention and reduce the primary symptoms associated with the precipitating event without following free associations that are unrelated to the target. He uses a modified EMDR (Mod-EMDR) script (see Chapter 20) that he has adapted from the EMD script; here, the target can be a single incident target memory or a representative worst memory from a group of memories related to the specific event. Russell reports using these scripts with patients after a near or immediate aftermath of exposure to a severe or potentially traumatic event or when patients present with severe acute stress responses or combat and operational stress reactions.

Elan Shapiro and Brurit Laub (2008) created a comprehensive protocol called "Recent Traumatic Episode Protocol" (R-TEP) that expands the existing protocols of EMD, ER-related protocols, and EMDR together and includes ways to contain and keep clients safe while processing. Their protocol introduces four important concepts: the Traumatic Episode, the Episode Narrative, the Google Search, and Telescopic Processing, all of which are discussed in Chapter 3.

R-TEP was used and research done with victims of a terrorist bombing in Gungoren, Istanbul (Altan Aytun et al., 2010). The participants were children and adults who scored high on the IES and the PTSD Symptom Checklist. R-TEP (incorporating EMD and Recent Event Protocols) was used with the adult participants who were seen weekly to work only on the trauma of the bombing; participants completed an IES prior to each session. The number of sessions was restricted to the completion of EMD and R-TEP. The data analyses demonstrate that EMDR was effective with the adults and helped in the prevention of PTSD and recommended the use of EMDR as a crisis intervention tool. The positive effect was maintained at a 3-month follow up. Tofani and Wheeler (2012) applied R-TEP in three different cases, observing markers such as distance concerning the trauma, a decrease in negative affect, access to information that is more adaptive, and changes in measures such as the SUDs, the VoC scale, and the revised IES-R, indicating changes in the perception of the traumatic memory. All three clients reported therapeutic changes in behavior and functioning. The EMDR R-TEP was used with over 2,000 survivors of recent earthquakes in northern Italy with pre- and posttreatment data collected showing changes in posttraumatic stress (Shapiro & Fernandez, 2013). Also, it was used with survivors from the recent earthquake in eastern Turkey in 2012 (Shapiro, 2012, p. 244).

Ignacio Jarero and Lucina Artigas created a different modification of Shapiro's (2001) Protocol for Recent Traumatic Events provided in an individual treatment format to clients suffering from recent ongoing trauma called the "EMDR Protocol for Recent Critical Incidents" (EMDR-PRECI). It was developed in the field under extremely dangerous circumstances to treat critical incidents where related stressful events continued for an extended time (often more than 6 months) and where there was no posttrauma period of safety for memory consolidation. Two randomized controlled trials (RCT) with the EMDR-PRECI have been published with delayed treatment designs supporting the efficacy of EMDR-PRECI in reducing symptoms after a 7.2 earthquake in North Baja California, Mexico (Jarero, Artigas, & Luber, 2011), and working with traumatized first responders responding to a human massacre situation (Jarero & Uribe, 2011, 2012).

An EMDR group protocol, the EMDR Integrative Group Treatment Protocol, was created in 1997 in Mexico after Hurricane Pauline (Artigas et al., 2000, 2009). Originally, this work was designed for children and combined the Standard EMDR Protocol with a group therapy model (Artigas et al., 2000; Jarero et al., 1999). However, it has been used with good success with disaster survivors from 7 years of age upward. There are a number of reports of its success worldwide (Aduriz, Knopfler, & Bluthgen, 2009; Errebo, Knipe, Forte, Karlin, & Altayli, 2008; Jarero et al., 2006, 2008), or with adaptations to meet the circumstances (Fernandez et al., 2004; Gelbach & Davis, 2007; Korkmazlar-Oral & Pamuk, 2002; Wilson, Tinker, Hofmann, Becker, & Marshall, 2000; Zaghrout-Hodali, Alissa, & Dodgson, 2008). Jarero and Artigas (2010) applied the EMDR-IGTP during 3 consecutive days to 20 adults in a Central American country with an ongoing geopolitical crisis. Results of this uncontrolled study showed decreases in scores on the SUDs and IES. Changes in the IES were maintained at a 14-week follow up even with the ongoing crisis. Louise Maxfield (2008, p. 75) wrote that, "EMDR-IGTP has been found effective in several field trials and has been used for thousands of disaster survivors around the world."

The Imma Protocol (2009, see Chapter 16) was adapted from the IGTP and includes the Four Elements for Stress Management (see Chapter 8) and group dynamic principles. Also, the Indian response team in Gujarat created an EMDR group protocol including the Butterfly Hug that was used with approximately 16,000 children in the area with positive results and decrease in traumatic symptoms.

There have been some cases described in the literature that discuss successful treatment of adults using EMD with two women, 1 month after the Great Hanshin-Awaji earthquake. They had been diagnosed with ASD. With both women, the SUDs decreased to 0 and the changes were maintained at a 5-month follow up (Ichii & Kumano, 1996).

Francine Shapiro's Protocol for Recent Traumatic Events was used with 9/11 survivors (Silver, Rogers, Knipe, & Colelli, 2005). They found that EMDR was a useful treatment intervention in the immediate aftermath of the event and later as well. In 2008, Colelli and Patterson found that their three cases demonstrated the usefulness of EMDR as a postdisaster treatment. It was only used in one case less than 3 months after 9/11; however, it was also found effective after 9 and 12 months. Fernandez (2002) used an average of 6.5 EMDR sessions for successful treatment with child survivors of the Molise earthquake in Italy; this was done over treatment cycles of 1 month, 3 months, and 1 year post incident. In 2008, Fernandez worked with a tsunami survivor diagnosed with acute PTSD and in a case study reported that after three EMDR sessions, the survivor was symptom free. The different forms of the EMDR protocol are being used quite actively in the EMDR community to relieve the distress of patients post disaster as has been previously illustrated. Given the amount of catastrophes that we seem to be facing in the world on a more and more regular basis, it is an appropriate time for a book such as *Implementing EMDR Early Mental Health Interventions for Man-Made and Natural Disasters: Models, Scripted Protocols, and Summary Sheets*.

The seed for *Implementing EMDR Early Mental Health Interventions for Man-Made and Natural Disasters: Models, Scripted Protocols, and Summary Sheets* grew out of this author's many exposures to recent trauma over the years: growing up under the constant threat of nuclear holocaust; living through the Vietnam era; hearing about sexual assault from my clients and about motor vehicle accidents; learning EMDR in 1992 and how to treat trauma-related issues; responding to Oklahoma City; training Israeli and Palestinian mental health practitioners to be EMDR facilitators and/or consultants and hearing their stories; meeting and working with trauma survivors of terrorist attacks in Jerusalem and Bethlehem; seeing the trauma symptoms displayed by Israeli supervisees during a supervisory course and working with their traumas after the second intifada; debriefing with the Philadelphia-based FBI group who responded to 9/11; assisting the friends and relatives of a friend after the brutal murder of his adolescent daughter; attending conferences where disaster responses were emphasized; interviewing 61 members of the EMDR community for the EMDRIA newsletter and hearing about their lives and how they have responded to many different types of disasters (i.e., hurricanes, earthquakes, terrorist attacks, war, acid attacks, etc.) in many different places (i.e., Oklahoma City, Bangladesh, New York, Serbia, Croatia,

Rwanda, Mexico, etc.); and talking and connecting with many more colleagues and friends after they returned from disaster responses.

In 2009, *Eye Movement Desensitization and Reprocessing (EMDR) Scripted Protocols: Basics and Special Situations* (Luber, 2009) was published. Although it was not a book about recent trauma per se, it did contain at least 10 out of 35 chapters that were recent-trauma related. Clearly, recent trauma was occupying this author's thoughts. This interest in recent trauma was amplified after a presentation at the EMDR European Annual Conference in Amsterdam. Konuk (2009, June) was presenting on *Mental Health Response and Training Program for Developing Countries: Turkish Model*. The depth and breadth of his response to this enormous natural disaster was inspiring and seemed an important model that other EMDR disaster responders would be interested to know about. This ongoing Turkish Project began with the response to the earthquake but was continuing currently, and he discussed the elements that he thought were pertinent to a disaster response: financing, the training of mental health professionals, providing psychological services, creating a trauma therapy center, building a trauma library, preparing for other disasters by engaging consultants who had experience in this area, and research. From 1999 until the time of the presentation (2009), his group trained 550 therapists in the EMDR Basic Training. They also trained 900 students and professionals in early trauma intervention skills. In the aftermath of their 1999 disaster project, the response teams have learned so much and are so well organized that they can be on-site within 30 to 60 minutes after any disaster in many areas in Turkey. As a result, they are held in high regard nationally and have had the ability to respond to more earthquakes, floods, bombings, and an airplane crash. *Emre's* pithy final words were the following, *"If you intend to go into the 'disaster business' in a developing country: Find the owner; find the money; teach organizational skills; teach how to write a proposal; and teach project management!"*

However, it was after the 2011 Tohoku earthquake and tsunami in Japan occurred that the need for this type of book became pressing. This author had visited Japan less than a year before the catastrophe to do an EMDR HAP Military training with Nancy Errebo at the Atsugi Naval Base several hours outside of Tokyo. In the hopes of supporting interaction between the EMDR Japan Association members and the American EMDR-trained mental health personnel on the U.S. military bases in Japan, this author made the formal introductions so that they could get to know and work with each other. When the disaster struck, we were all in touch with each other trying to find ways to support our Japanese colleagues. This author began to pull together the recent trauma-related protocols for our Japanese colleagues and helped them connect with other EMDR practitioners who were experts in the field of recent trauma—all of whom are represented in this book. It became clear that it would be far easier if all of these protocols were housed in one text and/or on a CD version; it was at that point that this author approached her editor at Springer Publishing Company, Sheri W. Sussman, with the idea. However, it was not just the protocols that were of importance; it was also how members of the EMDR community were responding to disasters globally. A proposal was written and accepted.

Implementing EMDR Early Mental Health Interventions for Man-Made and Natural Disasters: Models, Scripted Protocols, and Summary Sheets is akin to the structure in the other EMDR Scripted Protocol texts:

- *Eye Movement Desensitization and Reprocessing (EMDR) Scripted Protocols: Basics and Special Situations* (Luber, 2009a)
- *Eye Movement Desensitization and Reprocessing (EMDR) Scripted Protocols: Special Populations* (Luber, 2009b)
- *Eye Movement Desensitization and Reprocessing (EMDR) Scripted Protocols With Summary Sheets (CD-ROM Version)*: Basics and Special Situations (Luber, 2012a)
- *Eye Movement Desensitization and Reprocessing (EMDR) Scripted Protocols With Summary Sheets (CD-ROM Version): Special Populations* (Luber, 2012b)

The only exception to this structure is the inclusion of the first section on Early Mental Health Intervention Response: An International Perspective.

The following description from *Eye Movement Desensitization and Reprocessing (EMDR) Scripted Protocols: Basics and Special Situations* gives a clear understanding of the evolution and importance of this format:

> Eye Movement Desensitization and Reprocessing (EMDR) Scripted Protocols: Basics and Special Situations grew out of a perceived need that mental health practitioners could be served by a place to access both traditional and newly developed protocols in a way that adheres to best clinical practices incorporating the Standard EMDR Protocol that includes working on the past, present, and future issues (the 3-Pronged Protocol) related to the problem and the 11-Step Standard Procedure that includes attention to the following steps: image, negative cognition (NC), positive cognition (PC), validity of cognition (VoC), emotion, subjective units of disturbance (SUD), and location of body sensation, desensitization, installation, body scan, and closure. Often, EMDR texts embed the protocols in a great deal of explanatory material that is essential in the process of learning EMDR. However, sometimes, as a result, practitioners move away from the basic importance of maintaining the integrity of the Standard EMDR Protocol and keeping adaptive information processing in mind when conceptualizing the course of treatment for a patient. It is in this way that the efficacy of this powerful methodology is lost.
>
> "Scripting" becomes a way not only to inform and remind the EMDR practitioner of the component parts, sequence, and language used to create an effective outcome, but it also creates a template for practitioners and researchers to use for reliability and/or a common denominator so that the form of working with EMDR is consistent. The concept that has motivated this work was conceived within the context of assisting EMDR clinicians in accessing the scripts of the full protocols in one place and to profit from the creativity of other EMDR clinicians who have kept the spirit of EMDR but have also taken into consideration the needs of the population with whom they work or the situations that they encounter. Reading a script is by no means a substitute for adequate training, competence, clinical acumen, and integrity; if you are not a trained EMDR therapist and/or you are not knowledgeable in the field for which you wish to use the script, these scripts are not for you.
>
> As EMDR is a fairly complicated process, and indeed, has intimidated some from integrating it into their daily approach to therapy, this book provides step-by-step scripts that will enable beginning practitioners to enhance their expertise more quickly. . . .
>
> These scripted protocols are intended for clinicians who have read Shapiro's text (2001) and received EMDR training from an EMDR-accredited trainer. An EMDR trainer is a licensed mental health practitioner who has been approved by the association active in the clinician's country of practice. (Luber, 2009a, p. xxi)

In 2012, the CD-ROM versions of the original 2009 books were published in a different format. Included in the CD-ROM were just the protocols and summary sheets (the notes were not included and are in the 2009 texts). As explained in the Preface of *Eye Movement Desensitization and Reprocessing (EMDR) Scripted Protocols With Summary Sheets (CD-ROM Version): Basics and Special Situations* (Luber, 2012a):

> The idea for Eye Movement Desensitization and Reprocessing (EMDR) Scripted Protocols: Summary Sheets for Basics and Special Situations grew out of the day-to-day work with the protocols that allowed for a deeper understanding of case conceptualization from an EMDR perspective. While using the scripted protocols and acquiring a greater familiarity with the use of the content, the idea of placing the information in a summarized format grew. This book of scripted protocols and summary sheets was undertaken so that clinicians could easily use the material in Eye Movement Desensitization and Reprocessing (EMDR) Scripted Protocols: Basics and Special Situations. While working on the summary sheets, the interest in brevity collided with the thought that clinicians could also use these summary sheets to remind themselves of the steps in the process clarified in the scripted protocols. The original goal to be a summary of the necessary data gathered from the protocol was transformed into this new creation of data summary and memory tickler for the protocol itself! Alas, the summary sheets have become a bit longer than originally anticipated. Nonetheless, they are shorter—for the most part—than the protocols themselves and do summarize the data in an easily readable format. . . .
>
> The format for this book is also innovative. The scripts and summary sheets are available in an expandable, downloadable format for easy digital access. Because EMDR is a fairly complicated process, and often intimidating, these scripted protocols with their accompanying summary sheets can be helpful in a number of ways. To begin with, by facilitating the gathering of important

data from the protocol about the client, the scripted protocol and/or summary sheet then can be inserted into the client's chart as documentation. The summary sheet can assist the clinician in formulating a concise and clear treatment plan with clients and can be used to support quick retrieval of the essential issues and experiences during the course of treatment. Practitioners can enhance their expertise more quickly by having a place that instructs and reminds them of the essential parts of EMDR practice. By having these fill-in PDF forms, clinicians can easily tailor the scripted protocols and summary sheets to the needs of their clients, their consultees/supervisees, and themselves by editing and saving the protocol scripts and summary sheets.

Consultants/Supervisors will find these scripted protocols and summary sheets useful while working with consultees/supervisees in their consultation/supervision groups. These works bring together many ways of handling current, important issues in psychotherapy and EMDR treatment. They also include a helpful way to organize the data collected that is key to case consultation and the incorporation of EMDR into newly trained practitioners' practices. (Luber, 2012a, p. iv)

This main book is divided into eight parts with 26 chapters that include working with recent trauma models of response, resources, on-site responses, individuals, groups, special populations, special situations, and clinician self-care. The first part is devoted to the "Early Mental Health Intervention Response: An International Perspective." There are six chapters included in this section and all of them revolve around how disaster struck in the authors' environments and how they responded. Alan Cohen and Mooli Lahad explain the evolution of their Community Stress Prevention Center (CSPC) that was destined to become one of the earliest (1979)—if not *the* earliest—center to work with a mental health response in Israel and possibly in the world. Through the efforts of the CSPC, many people globally have learned how to respond to major disasters. Their influence is illustrated in the chapters from Turkey and Spain that follow. The second chapter is by Emre Konuk and his assistant, Zeynep Zat. As previously described above, Emre was part of the Turkish Psychological initiative to respond to the Marmara earthquake of 1999. They describe how, from the beginning, they incorporated a structure upon which they could improve their mental health disaster response capabilities over the years and then explain how they have gone on to accomplish it. Maria Cervera has been one of the major critical incident leaders in Spain. She describes how the Spanish psychologists—with the help of what they learned from Mooli Lahad's CSPC and the Independent Counseling and Advisory Services (ICAS)—built a national network of psychological professionals who are trained in mental health disaster response and related treatments. She explains a number of different interventions and how their ability to respond has made a difference throughout Spain. Ignacio (Nacho) Jarero and Susana Uribe take the opportunity in their chapter to describe Nacho's, "The Seven Phase Model." They describe this multicomponent model for an early psychological intervention program that is carried out by the Early Psychological Intervention Team (EPIT). They discuss in detail what to do before, during, and after deployment to the disaster zone. Through their organization, Asociación Mexicana Para Ayuda Mental en Crisis (AMAMECRISIS), they have assisted and taught their method to many clinicians. The fruits of their work—the Butterfly Hug, the EMDR Integrative Group Treatment Protocol (IGTP) for Children and for Adults, and the EMDR Protocol for Recent Critical Incidents (EMDR-PRECI)—are the gifts from them that we use all around the world. Carol Martin, the Executive Director of EMDR Humanitarian Assistance Programs (EMDR HAP), and Nancy Simons, Clinical Director of EMDR HAP, have written about the lessons learned by this program over the years. They go into more depth about the Trauma Recovery Networks (TRNs) that are forming across the United States to respond to local disasters in their communities and sometimes join other communities, if a response is needed. The last chapter in this part speaks to how a small group of volunteers from Mumbai were able to mount a huge response after the Gujarat earthquake of 2001. Sushma Mehrotra, Mrinalini Purandare, Parul Tank, and Hvovi Bhagwagar discuss this project and what they learned about responding to a major disaster. They, too, created an EMDR group protocol to respond to the needs of the victims.

The second part is devoted to "EMDR Early Mental Health Resources." Although there were many to choose from, there are only two of the most used resources in this section: the Butterfly Hug created by Luci Artigas and the Four Elements Exercise for Stress Management by Elan Shapiro. These two individuals have been central to the creation of a number of the chapters in this text, as a result of their sensitivity, creativity, and ability to transform a difficult situation by creating something totally new and specific to their context; they truly have the gift of turning therapy into an art form. "EMDR On-Site or Hospital Response" is the third section. In these chapters, we find very resourceful ways to work with trauma victims in the immediacy of their trauma. Gary Quinn's Emergency Response Procedure (ERP) gives us an important way to stabilize patients in the emergency room or on-site. Judith Guedalia's work assisted by Frances Yoeli is called the EMDR Emergency Room and Wards Protocol (EMDR-ER©) and they walk us through a thoughtful way of helping stabilize trauma survivors and creating new narratives for their trauma patients.

The fourth part, "EMDR Early Intervention Procedures for Individuals," presents the scripted protocol for Francine Shapiro's Protocol for Recent Traumatic Events, discussed in the beginning of this Preface. It is the basis—along with the Standard EMDR Protocol—upon which we have constructed our EMDR response for recent trauma. Elan Shapiro and Brurit Laub build on this foundation with their Recent Traumatic Episode Protocol (R-TEP) and help us conceptualize Early EMDR Intervention (EEI). Nacho Jarero and Luci Artigas end this section with their EMDR Protocol for Recent Critical Incidents (EMDR-PRECI). They, too, modify the Protocol for Recent Traumatic Events to incorporate the needs of the victims with whom they work.

"EMDR Early Intervention for Groups" is the subject of the fifth part. The first chapter is the ubiquitous, EMDR Integrative Group Treatment Protocol (IGTP) for Children and the second chapter is a newer version of the IGTP modified for adults. The IGTP has been the basis for group treatment since its inception in the late '90s and has been used around the world. The Imma EMDR Group Protocol by Brurit Laub and Esti Bar-Sade is a modification of the IGTP and offers some interesting and dynamic changes for working with children. Aiton Birnbaum is another creative individual who brought his talents to introducing a workbook format for EMDR. This new approach can be used with individuals or groups and can be helpful especially for those clients who are more visual. It also offers an option for a more private way of working with traumatic material. In this chapter, you will find an actual workbook that you can copy or print out for each client.

First responders are our society's designated protectors. Whether they are firefighters, emergency medical service professionals, the police, or the military, they are trained to respond when many of us would run in the other direction. In the first chapter of Part VI, "EMDR Early Mental Health Interventions: First Responders," Robbie Adler-Tapia delves into the world of first responders/protective service workers including firefighters and emergency medical services (EMS) professionals and helps us understand what we need to know to work with this population. Roger Solomon has been working with the police and law enforcement in many different capacities throughout the course of his career. He blends his knowledge of EMDR with his experience of the police to help us understand what we need to know to work with these officers of the law. Mark Russell is retired from the military with 26 years of service. He has translated his experience, with the help of his assistant, Tammera Cooke, and his colleague, Susan Rogers, a long-time provider of treatment to war and trauma survivors, to introduce us to the world of the military. All of these chapters introduce modifications when working with EMDR to accommodate the needs of first responders.

Part VII concerns "EMDR Early Intervention for Special Situations." The first chapter by David Blore is a protocol that addresses the particular issues regarding underground trauma. With his experience working with miners, David helps us enter into their domain so that we have a better appreciation for what the underground world is like and how to approach it when trauma strikes. The next chapter, which David wrote with Manda Holmshaw, grew out of his experience with clients who were uncomfortable revealing the content of their traumas and concerns. Through the EMDR "Blind to Therapist Protocol," they help clients reprocess their material with privacy and dignity.

The last section in the book, Part VIII, "EMDR and Clinician Self-Care: Recent Trauma Response," is at the heart of any well-designed disaster response. It is often the case that we take better care of our clients than ourselves. When it comes to disaster response, this attitude can be another type of disaster in the making. Neal Daniels's chapter discusses how we can inoculate ourselves against burnout and secondary PTSD by taking care to process residual material from our work on a regular basis. In Karen Alter-Reid's chapter about her own FR-TRN response to the Newtown shooting tragedy, self-care is a primary ingredient in the organization of their work. There are a number of checks and support systems that create a holding environment for the team so that no one slips through the cracks to face the aftermath of disaster response alone. Derek Farrell responded to the call for facilitators and volunteers to assist in Turkey after the earthquake. His chapter teaches us about how even the most perceptive of clinicians can miss something in the face of such overwhelming destruction. Derek teaches us the signs and symptoms of vicarious trauma and then uses this knowledge to create better caretaking for himself and his clients. The last chapter in this section and the book is about the worst case scenarios in recent trauma response. Nacho and Susana again use the format that they did in Chapter 4 of pre-, during, and post-deployment to create checklists to assure that you have thought of all the variables when responding to disaster.

Appendix A includes the scripts for the 3-Pronged Protocol that includes past memories, current triggers, and future templates. These scripts are there to assist practitioners so that they can place them in clients' charts to use with a particular issue or as a reminder of all of the elements needed for the work to be complete.

Appendix B is an updated list of all of the EMDR associations and regional associations globally. In this way, it is possible to know where practitioners of EMDR are to be found in any part of the world. This list also includes the EMDR Humanitarian Assistance Programs that exist to help victims of man-made and natural disasters. There are also resources that catalogue information such as the Francine Shapiro Library, an invaluable source of knowledge for any EMDR practitioner. There are also links to the *EMDR Journal* and other e-journals where trauma-related information can be found.

This book is meant to go with you to disasters. Here, you will find a great deal of information that will support you in responding to the challenges that you might face when designing a disaster response or responding to a disaster. Each one of these protocols has been tried in the field. Although there is no definitive research about them, it has begun to trickle in, and you can be the next author of research in this area. Try these suggestions and protocols in your own community and join your Humanitarian Assistance Program groups and/or TRNs to create an EMDR disaster response that is felt around the world.

REFERENCES

Aduriz, M. E., Knopfler, C., & Bluthgen, C. (2009). Helping child flood victims using group EMDR intervention in Argentina: Treatment outcome and gender differences. *International Journal of Stress Management, 16*, 138–153.

Altan Aytun, O., Ozcan, G., Ciftci, A,. Konuk, E., Yuksek, H., Karakus, D., . . . Vatan Ozcelik, D. (2010, June). The effects of early EMDR interventions (EMD and R-TEP) on the victims of a terrorist bombing in Istanbul. In *Treatment of children/acute stress*. Symposium conducted at the annual meeting of the EMDR Europe Association, Hamburg, Germany.

American Psychiatric Association (APA). (2004). *Practice guideline for the treatment of patients with acute stress disorder and posttraumatic stress disorder*. Arlington, VA: American Psychiatric Association Practice Guidelines.

Andrews, B., Brewin, C. R., Philpott, R., & Stewart, L. (2007). Delayed-onset posttraumatic stress disorder: A systematic review of the evidence. *American Journal of Psychiatry, 164*(9), 1319–1326.

Artigas, L., Jarero, I., Mauer, M., López Cano, T., & Alcalá, N. (2000, September). *EMDR and traumatic stress after natural disasters: Integrative treatment protocol and the Butterfly Hug*. Poster presented at the EMDRIA Conference, Toronto, Ontario, Canada.

Artigas, L., Jarero, I., Alcalá, N., & Lopez-Cano, T. (2009). The EMDR Integrative Group Treatment Protocol (IGTP). In M. Luber (Ed.), *Eye movement desensitization and reprocessing (EMDR) scripted protocols: Basic and special situations* (pp. 279–288). New York, NY: Springer.

Australian Centre for Posttraumatic Mental Health. (2007). *Australian guidelines for the treatment of adults with acute stress disorder and posttraumatic stress disorder*. Melbourne, Victoria: Author.

Bleich, A., Kotler, M., Kutz, I., & Shalev, A. (2002). *Guidelines for the assessment and professional intervention with terror victims in the hospital and in the community*. A position paper of the (Israeli) National Council for Mental Health, Jerusalem, Israel.

Bryant, R. A., Creamer, M., O'Donnell, M., Silove, D., & McFarlane, A. C. (2011). The capacity of acute stress disorder to predict posttraumatic psychiatric disorders. *Journal of Psychiatric Research, 46*(2), 168–173.

Bryant, R. A., Friedman, M. J., Spiegel, D., Ursano, R., & Strain. J. (2010). A review of acute stress disorder in *DSM-5*. *Depression and Anxiety, 28*(9), 802–817.

California Evidence-Based Clearinghouse for Child Welfare. (2010). *Trauma treatment for children*. Retrieved from www.cebc4cw.org

Chambless, D. L., Baker, M. J., Baucom, D. H., Beutler, L. E., Calhoun, K. S., Cris-Christoph, P., . . . Woody, S. R. (1998). Update on empirically validated therapies, II. *The Clinical Psychologist, 51*, 3–16.

Chemtob, C. M., Tolin, D. F., van der Kolk, B. A., & Pitman, R. K. (2000). Eye movement desensitization and reprocessing. In E. A. Foa, T. M. Keane, & M. J. Friedman (Eds.), *Effective treatments for PTSD: Practice guidelines from the International Society for Traumatic Stress Studies*. New York, NY: Guilford.

Clinical Resource Efficiency Support Team. (2003). *The management of posttraumatic stress disorder in adults*. A publication of the Clinical Resource Efficiency Support Team of the Northern Ireland Department of Health, Social Services and Public Safety, Belfast.

Colelli, G., & Patterson, B. (2008). Three case reports illustrating the use of the Protocol for Recent Traumatic Events following the World Trade Center terrorist attack. *Journal of EMDR Practice and Research, 2*(2), 114–123.

Department of Veterans Affairs and Department of Defense. (2004). *VA/DoD clinical practice guideline for the management of post-traumatic stress*. Washington, DC: Veterans Health Administration, Department of Veterans Affairs and Health Affairs, Department of Defense. Office of Quality and Performance publication 10Q-CPG/PTSD-04.

Dutch National Steering Committee Guidelines Mental Health Care. (2003). *Multidisciplinary guideline anxiety disorders*. Utrecht, Netherlands: Quality Institute Health Care CBO/Trimbos Institute.

Errebo, N., Knipe, J., Forte, K., Karlin, V., & Altayli, B. (2008). EMDR-HAP training in Sri Lanka following 2004 tsunami. *Journal of EMDR Practice & Research, Fernandez (2002), 2*(2), 124–139.

Fernandez, I. (2002, Dicembre). I disturbi post-traumatici da stress Fattori di rischio, aspetti diagnostici e trattamento con l'EMDR (The post-traumatic stress disorder factors of risk, diagnostic aspects and treatment with the EMDR). *Rivista Scientifica di Psicologia, Sommario 01*, 15–124.

Fernandez, I. (2007). EMDR as treatment of post-traumatic reactions: A field study on children victims of an earthquake. *Educational and Child Psychology, 24*(1), 65–72.

Fernandez, I. (2008). EMDR after a critical incident: Treatment of a tsunami survivor with acute posttraumatic disorder. *Journal of EMDR Practice and Research, 2*(2), 156–159.

Fernandez, I., Gallinari, E., & Lorenzetti, A. (2004). A school-based intervention for children who witnessed the Pirelli building airplane crash in Milan, Italy. *Journal of Brief Therapy, 2*, 129–136.

Foa, E. B. (2009). *Effective treatments for PTSD: Practice guidelines from the International Society for Traumatic Stress Studies* (2nd ed.). New York, NY: Guilford.

Gelbach, R., & Davis, K. (2007). Disaster response: EMDR and family systems therapy under community-wide stress. In F. Shapiro, F. W. Kaslow, & L. Maxfield (Eds.), *Handbook of EMDR and family therapy processes* (pp. 387–406). New York, NY: John Wiley.

Grainger, R. D., Levin, C., Allen-Byrd, L., Doctor, R. M., & Lee, H. (1997). An empirical evaluation of eye movement desensitization and reprocessing (EMDR) with survivors of a natural disaster. *Journal of Traumatic Stress, 10*, 665–671.

Ichii, M., & Kumano, H. (1996a). Application of eye movement desensitization (EMD) to the acute stress disorder victims suffered from the Great Hanshin-Awaji earthquake. *Japanese Journal of Brief Psychotherapy, 5*, 53–68.

Ichii, M., & Kumano, H. (1996b). Eye movement desensitization by Kobe earthquake victims with acute stress disorder (EMD) application. *Japanese Association of Brief Psychotherapy, Research Brief, 5*, 53–70.

INSERM. (2004). *Psychotherapy: An evaluation of three approaches*. Paris, France: French National Institute of Health and Medical Research.

Jarero, I., & Artigas, L. (2010). The EMDR Integrative Group Treatment Protocol: Application with adults during ongoing geopolitical crisis. *Journal of EMDR Practice and Research, 4*(4), 148–155.

Jarero, I., Artigas, L., & Hartung, J. (2006). EMDR Integrative Group Treatment Protocol: A post-disaster trauma intervention for children and adults. *Traumatology, 12*, 121–129.

Jarero, I., Artigas, L., & Luber, M. (2011). The EMDR Protocol for Recent Critical Incidents: Application in a disaster mental health continuum of care context. *Journal of EMDR Practice and Research, 5*(3), 82–94.

Jarero, I., Artigas, L., Mauer, M., López Cano, T., & Alcalá, N. (1999, November). *Children's post traumatic stress after natural disasters: Integrative treatment protocol*. Poster presented at the annual meeting of the International Society for Traumatic Stress Studies, Miami, Florida.

Jarero, I., Artigas, L., & Montero, M. (2008). The EMDR Integrative Group Treatment Protocol: Application with child victims of mass disaster. *Journal of EMDR Practice & Research, 2*(2), 97–105.

Jarero, I., & Uribe, S. (2011). The EMDR Protocol for Recent Critical Incidents: Brief report of an application in a human massacre situation. *Journal of EMDR Practice and Research, 5*(4), 156–165.

Jarero, I., & Uribe, S. (2012). The EMDR Protocol for Recent Critical Incidents: Follow-up report of an application in a human massacre situation. *Journal of EMDR Practice and Research, 6*(2), 50–61.

Korkmazlar-Oral, U., & Pamuk, S. (2002). Group EMDR with child survivors of the earthquake in Turkey. *Journal of the American Academy of Child and Adolescent Psychiatry, 37*, 47–50.

Konuk, E. (June, 2009). *Mental health response and training program for developing countries: Turkish model*. Paper presented at the EMDR Europe Association Conference, Amsterdam.

Kutz, I., Resnick, V., & Dekel, R. (2008). The effect of single-session modified EMDR on acute stress syndromes. *Journal of EMDR Practice and Research, 2*(3), 190–200.

Laub, B., & Bar-Sade, E. (2009a). In M. Luber (Ed.), *Eye movement desensitization and reprocessing (EMDR) scripted protocols: Basics and special situations*. New York, NY: Springer.

Luber, M. (Ed.). (2009a). *Eye movement desensitization and reprocessing (EMDR) scripted protocols: Basics and special situations*. New York, NY: Springer.

Luber, M. (Ed.). (2009b). *Eye movement desensitization and reprocessing (EMDR) scripted protocols: Special populations*. New York, NY: Springer.

Luber, M. (Ed.). (2012a). *Eye movement desensitization and reprocessing (EMDR) scripted protocols with summary sheets (CD-ROM version): Basics and special situations*. New York, NY: Springer.

Luber, M. (Ed.). (2012b). *Eye movement desensitization and reprocessing (EMDR) scripted protocols with summary sheets (CD-ROM version): Special populations*. New York, NY: Springer.

Maxfield, L. (2008). EMDR treatment of recent events and community disasters. *Journal of EMDR Practice & Research, 2*(2), 74–78.

McFarlane, A. C. (2010a). *Abstract to plenary presentation*. Paper presented at EMDR Europe Annual Conference, Hamburg, Germany.

McFarlane, A. C. (2010b). The long-term costs of traumatic stress: Intertwined physical and psychological consequences. *World Psychiatry, 9*, 3–10.

National Collaborating Centre for Mental Health. (2005). *Post traumatic stress disorder (PTSD): The management of adults and children in primary and secondary care*. London, England: National Institute for Clinical Excellence.

National Institute for Clinical Excellence. (2005, March). *Post-traumatic stress (PTSD): The management of PTSD in adults and children and secondary care*. London, England: National Collaborating Centre for Mental Health.

Roberts, N. P., Kitchiner, N. J., Kenardy, J., & Bisson, J. I. (2009). Multiple session early psychological interventions for the prevention of post-traumatic stress disorder. *The Cochrane Library* (Issue 3). [DOI: 10.1002/14651858.CD006869.pub2].

Roberts, N. P., Kitchiner, N. J., Kenardy, J., & Bisson, J. I. (2009). Systematic review and meta-analysis of multiple-session early interventions following traumatic events. *American Psychiatric Association, AJP in Advance*. Retrieved from ajp.psychiatryonline.org

Russell, M. C. (2006). Treating combat-related stress disorders: Multiple case study utilizing eye movement desensitization and reprocessing (EMDR) with battlefield casualties from the Iraqi war. *Military Psychology, 18*, 1–18.

SAMHSA's National Registry of Evidence-Based Programs and Practices. (2011). Retrieved from http://nrepp.samhsa.gov/ViewIntervention.aspx?id=199

Schubert, S., & Lee, C. W. (2009). Adult PTSD and its treatment with EMDR: A review of controversies, evidence, and theoretical knowledge. *Journal of EMDR Practice and Research, 3*(3), 117–132.

Shapiro, E. (2009). EMDR treatment of recent trauma. *Journal of EMDR Practice and Research, 3*(3), 141–151.

Shapiro, E. (2012, October). EMDR and early psychological intervention following trauma. *European Review of Applied Psychology, 62*(4), 241–251.

Shapiro, E., & Fernandez, I. (2013, June). *Early EMDR intervention (EEI): Theory, practice and research application in a mass disaster*. Presentation at the annual meeting of the EMDR Europe Association, Geneva, Switzerland.

Shapiro, E., & Laub, B. (2008). Early EMDR intervention (EEI): A summary, a theoretical model, and the recent traumatic episode protocol (R-TEP). *Journal of EMDR Practice and Research, 2*(2), 79–96.

Shapiro, F. (1989). Eye movement desensitization: A new treatment model for post-traumatic stress disorder. *Journal of Behavior Therapy and Experimental Psychiatry, 20*, 211–217.

Shapiro, F. (1991). Eye movement desensitization and reprocessing procedure: From EMD to EMDR-a new treatment model for anxiety and related traumata. *Behavior Therapist, 14*, 122–125.

Shapiro, F. (1995). *Eye movement desensitization and reprocessing: Basic principles, protocols and procedures*. New York, NY: Guilford Press.

Shapiro, F. (2001). *Eye movement desensitization and reprocessing: Basic principles, protocols and procedures* (2nd ed.). New York, NY: Guilford Press.

Shapiro, F. (2004). *Military and post-disaster response manual*. Hamden, CT: EMDR Humanitarian Assistance Program.

Shapiro, F. (2006). *EMDR: New notes on adaptive information processing with case formulation principles, forms, scripts and worksheets*. Watsonville, CA: EMDR Institute.

Shapiro, F., Kaslow, F. W., & Maxfield, L. (2007). *Handbook of EMDR and family therapy processes*. Hoboken, NJ: Wiley.

Silver, S. M., Rogers, S., Knipe, J., & Colelli, G. (2005, February). EMDR therapy following the 9/11 terrorist attacks: A community-based intervention project in New York City. *International Journal of Stress Management, 12*(1), 29–42.

Sjöblom, P. O., Andréewitch, S., Bejerot, S., Mörtberg, E., Brinck, U., Ruck, C., & Körlin, D. (2003). *Regional treatment recommendation for anxiety disorders*. Stockholm, Sweden: Medical Program Committee/Stockholm

Therapy Advisor. (2004–2007), Retrieved from www.therapyadvisor.com

Tofani, L. R., & Wheeler, K. (2012). Le protocole de l'épisode traumatique récent: Evaluation et analyse des résultats de trois études de cas [The protocol for recent traumatic episode: Evaluation and analysis of the results of three case studies]. *Journal of EMDR Practice and Research, 6*(4), 46E–63E.

United Kingdom Department of Health. (2001). *Treatment choice in psychological therapies and counselling evidence based clinical practice guideline*. London, England: Author.

U.S. Department of Veterans Affairs, Veterans Health Administration & Department of Defense. (2004, January). VA/DoD clinical practice guideline for the management of post-traumatic stress. Version 1.0. Washington, DC: Veterans Health Administration, and Department of Defense.

Vanitallie, T. B. (2002). Stress: A risk factor for serious illness. *Metabolism, 51*(6 Suppl. 1), 40–45.

Wesson, M., & Gould, M. (2009). Intervening early with EMDR on military operations. *Journal of EMDR Practice and Research, 3*(2), 91–97.

Wilson, S., Tinker, R., Hofmann, A., Becker, L., & Marshall, S. (2000). *A field study of EMDR with Kosovar-Albanian refugee children using a group treatment protocol*. Paper presented at the annual meeting of the International Society for the Study of Traumatic Stress, San Antonio, TX.

Zaghrout-Hodali, M., Alissa, F., & Dodgson, P. (2008). Building resilience and dismantling fear: EMDR group protocol with children in an area of ongoing trauma. *Journal of EMDR Practice & Research, 2*(2), 106–113.

Acknowledgments

As a young girl and on into my adolescence, I had the good fortune to grow up in an international community. In this oasis of the International School of Geneva (Ecolint) and under the greater global community fostered by the many international organizations that were headquartered there, I lived in a place where we all coexisted in a type of harmony that—it turns out—is rare. Our school community had its wrinkles but the bullying and the rage that one hears so frequently now, at least to me, was not apparent. We learned to think and reason and negotiate. Through our Students' United Nations, we fought the battles of our world through words and compromise. Simply put, we all got along with each other and if we had a problem, we worked it out. My first year of college shattered that pristine experience of cooperation and tolerance; it was 1968 and the end of my first year when the streets of Paris erupted and chaos ensued as "La revolution de mai" held the whole city hostage. Returning to the States in the middle of the Vietnam War opened my eyes to the fact that the lessons that I learned in Geneva were certainly not happening where I found myself and I discovered later that my friends from Ecolint felt that same way. Since then, I have learned a great deal about trauma and, sadly, it is everywhere.

I would like to acknowledge the need for us—as an EMDR international community—to be part of an initiative to turn this state of affairs around. This book, *Implementing EMDR Early Mental Health Interventions for Man-Made and Natural Disasters: Models, Scripted Protocols, and Summary Sheets*, is an attempt to help my colleagues in the EMDR community learn more about what is needed to respond in the face of disaster and help victims heal and reclaim their lives.

I had two major experiences that pushed me toward the formulation of this book: hearing Emre Konuk present and the 2011 Tōhoku earthquake and tsunami in Japan. First, I would like to acknowledge my friend and colleague, Emre Konuk. It was Emre's presentation at the 2009 EMDR Europe Conference on the Turkish Model for a mental health response that inspired me to learn more about disaster response. As I got to know Emre better through attending conferences and a trip to Turkey, I heard more and more about the breadth and depth of his projects and felt that his gift of organization and creating projects for the greater good was information that we all needed to access.

The 2011 disaster in Japan was of a more personal nature for me. I first traveled to Japan in 1976 with my parents, who had a small business selling Japanese prints. I opened a Japanese art gallery that same year with my father and for a short time I ran the gallery before I decided to go back to teaching and then become a clinical psychologist. The gallery continued and the walls of my world have literally been filled with the aesthetic of Japan since then. I have been back several more times since my first trip for personal, art, and EMDR-related work.

I would like to acknowledge the work of Masaya Ichii who—in fact—was one of the first to use EMD with earthquake survivors after the 1995 Kobe earthquake. Masaya has gone on to become a trainer and create J-HAP, and has been an important force in helping EMDR develop in Japan. I would also like to acknowledge Shigeyuki Ota who did much to support the Japanese response in Tōhoku, as well as Elan Shapiro, Brurit Laub, Nacho Jarero, Masamichi Honda, Kiwamu Tanaka, Masako Kitamura, Robert Gelbach, Derek Farrell, Sushma Mehrotra, Richard Smith, Emre Konuk, Miyako Shirakawa, Akiko Kikuchi,

Keisuki Niki, Pam Brown, Rashid Qayyum, and many other EMDR colleagues from all over the world who helped sustain the EMDR response in Japan.

From the early days of EMDR, Roger Solomon's name was synonymous with working in the area of recent trauma. With his knowledge and experience with the police and other law enforcement agencies, Roger was the person to whom we all went when we had questions concerning early EMDR intervention, critical incident response, and traumatic grief. I would like to acknowledge Roger for all of the work that he has done in this area for all of us in the EMDR community. I would also like to thank you for your support over the years and the grace with which you answered all the questions that I had or assisted me with your insights concerning areas of recent trauma, no matter where you were or what you were doing. Also, for reconnecting me with my old friend, Jim McIntosh, who as an FBI agent helped me understand more clearly the impact of recent trauma and the horrors of 9/11.

I would like us all to remember and celebrate Jim who passed away after his own long battle with illness for his service to his family, friends, and country.

I would like to recognize my friend, Robert Wittman, fellow traveler, FBI agent, and Japanese aficionado who always knows how to climb over any mountain to get to the other side.

There are a number of other people whom I would like to acknowledge concerning this book as it would not have happened without the learning that I gained from our discussions; the hashing out and back and forth of our conversations helped me have a greater appreciation for the nuances of these ideas. To my friends, Elan Shapiro and Brurit Laub, words cannot express how much our discussions have meant to me in the understanding of early EMDR intervention and my respect for your continuing creativity and kindness of spirit. To the three gentleman who underwrote my "trauma fact-finding trip" to Kiryat Schmona (Alan Cohen), Jerusalem (Gary Quinn), and Tel Aviv (Udi Oren) to help me understand the impact of recent trauma and find ways to raise money for more EMDR trainings in the Middle East. To all of the consultants who attended the many consultancy trainings that we (often with Elan) created together in Israel—your willingness to share the innermost parts of yourselves during our work together created a profound learning experience that touched me deeply.

I would like to acknowledge Nacho Jarero, Lucy Artigas, and Susana Uribe—a braver group of people I cannot imagine. Thank you for your friendship and the joy that you take in the most simple of pleasures, even as you go into "battle" or put on your hazmat suits. I have learned more about the spirit that one needs to face the evils of the world and come out on the other side well and—always—with the "Ministry of Presence."

I would like to acknowledge the strength and heart of my female friends and colleagues: Lucy Artigas, Sushma Mehrotra, Mona Zaghrout, Maria Cervera, Robbie Dunton, Rosalie Thomas, Peggy Moore, Susanna Uribe, Kerstin Bergh Johannesson, Phyllis Klaus, Zara Yellin, Zona Scheiner, Barbara Hensley, Catherine Fine, Irene Geissl, Elaine Alvarez, Barbara Grinnell, Robbie Adler-Tapia, Carolyn Settle, Kate Wheeler, Sandra Wilson, Victoria Britt, Sheila Bender, Marsha Heiman, Delphine Pecoul, Maria Elena Aduriz, Ligia Barascout de Piedra Santa, Louise Maxfield, Joany Spierings, Reyhana Ravat, Jennifer Lendl, Deany Laliotis, Francisca Garcia Guerra, Esly Carvalho, Eva Muenker-Kramer, Nancy Errebo, Luise Reddemann, Phyllis Goltra, Priscilla Marquis, Barbara Parrett, Carlijn de Roos, Linda Cohn, Jocelyne Shiromoto, Christine Rost, Martine Tiedt-Schutte, Elfrun Magloire, Eva Zimmerman, Esther Ebner, France Haour, Hanne Hummel, Shelley Weber, Hope Riley, Brenda Byrne, Veronika Engl, Isabel Fernancez, Sandy Shapiro, Ruth Heber, Ellen Latenstein, Karen Alter Reid, Sue Evans, Susan Schaefer, Lulu Medina, Debby Korn, Brurit Laub, Sandra Wilson, Elizabeth Snyker, Hellen Hornsveld, Renee Beer, Christie Sprowls, Barbara Korzun, Patti Levin, Jocelyn Barrett, Reg Morrow, Carol Crow, Carol Forgash, Esti Bar Sade, Isabelle Meignant, Tessa Prattos, Jenny Ann Rydberg, Fran Yoeli, Katy Murray, Sandra Paulsen, Donna D'Aloia, Katy O'Shea, Sandra Kaplan, Nancy Smith, Dorothy Ashman, Wendy Freitag, Pam Brown, Laurie Tetrault, Ana Gomez, Kay Werk, Debra Wesselmann, Maria Masciandaro, Betsy Prince, Jill Strunk, Denise Gelinas, Sandi Richman, Shelley Uram, Frankie Klaff, Edith Taber, Celia Grand, Cynthia Kong, Blanche Freund, Francine Shapiro, and all of the extraordinary women I have met on this journey.

To Derek Farrell who has become a friend—not just a colleague—over the past several years, I would like to thank you for your ability to keep grounded despite the difficulties around you and for the gift of your experience that you have given to all of us.

To Richard Mitchell, my old friend and fellow voyager on our trip to Bethlehem that opened our eyes and souls. To Jim Knipe who has been a great support. To Bob Gelbach, Howard Wainer, Donald Nathanson, and Stuart Wolfe who have been strong supporters of my writing. To AJ Popky who introduced me to EMDR.

To Steve Silver, I thank you for all that I have learned from you while doing EMDR supervision groups together, for your willingness to answer questions, and for always looking for the "light in the heart of darkness." I would like to acknowledge Susan Rogers and Elaine Alvarez for stepping in at a time that I needed assistance and making everything clear. Thank you also to Elan Shapiro, Brurit Laub, Nacho Jarero, and Roger Solomon for helping when another set of eyes or four was needed.

I would also like to remember Kathy Davis who left us with the legacy of her wisdom, her knowledge, and her kindness.

I would like to thank the Springer staff, especially my editor, Sheri W. Sussman, for her encouragement and support in the face of many demands on my time during this period of writing.

Always, I want to thank and acknowledge you, Francine. Your discovery, your creativity, your persistence, and your ability to open a new door that is EMDR has been one of the greatest gifts in my life and uncountable others.

I am dedicating this book to my mother who has been going through her own recent trauma with the spirit and true determination that she has always displayed throughout her life; a role model for us all.

EMDR On-Site or Hospital Response

In the chaos that ensues after any type of catastrophe, the pain and suffering of people rends our hearts. Working under these circumstances—as most first responders do—takes a certain kind of resiliency and dedication. In this section, the authors have chosen to work in the emergency rooms in hospitals. Each chapter has its own perspective on treating the victims who are usually carried through the doors, often screaming, yelling, in shock, staring blankly, eyes forward, disoriented, and/or in panic. Often, they are followed by their friends and/or family—who were with them—or had found out that they had been taken to the hospital. They, too, are in various degrees of shock, fear, anger, and/or distress.

The first order of business is the patient's physical needs. It is usually after these are met that mental health providers can assume a role in the patient's care. Gary Quinn is a medical doctor who lives in Jerusalem and has been concerned about the welfare of those who have been traumatized by terrorist attacks, military trauma, and motor vehicle accidents. He is in private practice and earlier in his EMDR career began volunteering his time to help trauma survivors in the emergency room. In his chapter, the "Emergency Response Procedure (ERP)," Gary teaches us a way to respond to patients when they have been just brought into the ER. Over the years, Gary and other colleagues have used the ERP during initial hospitalizations, critical incident scenes, when an abreaction occurs during the history or preparation phases of EMDR, and as a cognitive interweave, as well as in the ER. Gary's approach for the most part is to help the patient jumpstart the self-regulatory system that comes from realizing the danger is over and that she is safe in the present.

Judith Guedalia has been the senior medical psychologist and a member of the emergency room trauma staff, where she has responded to more than 26 mass casualty events (MCEs). Over the years, she has crafted a particular way to respond to patients under her care. Her friend and colleague, Frances Yoeli, headed the Emergency Mental Health Team in the Emek Bet-Shean for many years. Their chapter, "EMDR Emergency Room and Wards Protocol (EMDR-ER©)," grew out of Judith's work under these circumstances, and Fran contributed her knowledge of EMDR to support the inclusion of this method into Judith's way of approaching patients in the ERs and wards after MCEs. Their patients often spend 5 to 8 hours in the ER, allowing them to layer in an EMDR response in an interesting manner. Once the patient reaches a basic level of safety and trust with the therapist and is more oriented, the EMDR-ER© is possible. This protocol is not to be used with people who are showing signs of hysterical paralysis or fugue-like states or with patients with below borderline intelligences as EMDR may be too stimulating for them at this time. By making the rounds of the patients who may often number into the double digits, they keep returning to each patient, asking again for their narrative and taking notes. In this way, they are performing a form of titrated review, allowing for the dilution of the emotion that accompanies their recollection, while weaving in first the positive cognition to help affirm the issues of safety, control, and recovery and using positive acts of kindness or positive experiences patients referred to in their narratives while using BLS, if possible, to create new narratives of the experiences.

Both of these models of early intervention have much to offer the clinician working in the immediacy of the emergency room or any other critical care scenario. Each chapter includes a summary sheet for data entry and to remind you of the steps of these protocols. Prepared with this type of knowledge, the mental health practitioner can be an asset to any early response.

Emergency Response Procedure (ERP)

Gary Quinn

Introduction

The Emergency Response Procedure (ERP) was initially developed to help victims within hours of a terrorist attack, but can be applied in the minutes and hours following any trauma. Often, at that time, the patient has difficulty in orienting to the present after having experienced danger to self, family, or friends. When the clinician reorients a person to their present state of safety with ERP, he is assisting in a crucial task of adaptation by helping the victim's brain to understand that the danger has passed and the person is safe in the present.

The goal of ERP is to support patients in recognizing that they are "safe now" from the trauma that has just occurred. The incident is in the past and they can resume a present time orientation, as evidenced by calmer behavior and the ability to communicate verbally. If patients remain nonverbal, further intervention (including additional ERP) is immediately indicated.

The Emergency Response Procedure is versatile and has been utilized in the following locations and situations:

- Emergency room
- During initial hospitalization
- Immediate intervention in communal distress centers
- Critical incident scenes such as car accidents, earthquakes, natural or human-made disasters, death of a loved one, and in ambulances
- Abreaction during the initial history taking, prior to the Preparation Phase of EMDR
- During EMDR, and at other times when patients appear to be deeply fearful, it can be used as an interweave, to return them to a sense of present-time safety

Critical Incident Responses and ERP

Normally, after a critical incident, individuals present with a wide range of responses as reported in the Subjective Units of Disturbance (SUD) scale, where 0 = no disturbance and 10 = the highest disturbance possible. The individuals who arrive in emergency rooms/centers just after a critical incident usually report a SUDs of 7–10+ /10. These victims are suffering greatly and are in need of immediate intervention to assist them in calming and deescalating.

Note: It is possible that this group later moves from an Acute Stress Reaction (ASR) to an Acute Stress Disorder (ASD). According to Briere and Scott (2006, p.166), 80% of those whose symptoms are initially severe enough to meet criteria for ASD will have PTSD six months later, while 60–70% will still have PTSD two years following the event.

Although it is possible that those patients with a 3–7/10 score could benefit from ERP, this group often is able to self-soothe. Therefore, more efficient use of the ERP practitioner's time will be with patients in a "highly agitated" state (7–10/10), and those who have moved into a "silent terror" (10 + /10).

"Highly Agitated State:" When a patient is in a highly agitated state, her internal self-regulating system is not able to turn down the activation mechanisms, after the experience of danger has passed. When the sympathetic nervous system is activated, individuals will show symptoms including crying, screaming, yelling that they are not safe, increased arousal, irritability, poor concentration, hypervigilance, exaggerated startle response, motor restlessness, and an inability to execute necessary tasks. They are never silent. They are conspicuous to emergency staff because of their excessive noise. Not yet realizing they are safe from the event, these individuals are rarely able to present a coherent story and often act as though they remain in the middle of a dangerous situation.

In a sense, ERP jumpstarts the patient's self-regulatory system to reset and return to a state of calm that naturally occurs once the danger is over. Behavioral indicators of this relatively calmed state may include:

- Orienting to the present
- Interacting with first responders, family, and friends
- Inquiring as to family member whereabouts
- Talking about leaving the treatment location
- Discussing next steps and discharge arrangements
- Considering feasible living arrangements if needed

"Silent Terror" State: Beyond the "highly agitated state," patients may present with silent terror characterized by a dazed appearance, shaking and/or the inability to speak. Those experiencing silent terror have a 10 + score on the SUD scale. During a traumatic event, the sympathetic nervous system produces a normal response to danger of "fight or flight." However, when a person cannot fight or escape, the parasympathetic system kicks in and produces the "freeze" or silent terror response.

ERP is as effective for this group as it is for individuals presenting in a highly agitated state. Originally, when working with those in silent terror, this author believed that the ERP would not be helpful. These were the patients who were often ignored during an active rescue scene since they were silent. They would simply lie on the ground or on their stretchers and appear not to be suffering, much like patients immediately after surgery. Mistakenly, these patients were thought not to require immediate intervention.

While working on-site with patients, this author chanced using ERP with several individuals who were exhibiting silent terror. The true positive cognition, *"You are safe now,"* was employed and accompanied by bilateral stimulation. Later, when these patients were able to speak, they reported that although they did not seem to respond to what was said to them, many were actually enduring repeated flashbacks of the recently concluded traumatic event. They reported being terribly frightened and trapped in their inability to communicate with anyone about it.

Following administration of ERP, they began to speak and exhibit behaviors similar to those in the highly agitated group. This author continued saying, *"You are safe and now in the ER and you are okay,"* until their agitation calmed down. In subsequent debriefings, these patients came to realize that during their silent terror they were in a highly agitated state, but were incapable of telling anyone; thus, the term, silent terror.

ERP administered at these times seemed to re-engage the Adaptive Information Processing system. Once the recent danger was over, patients' AIP systems were unblocked and able to process the reality that they were "safe now." The activated system was able to return to normal.

Emergency Response Procedure Script Notes

ERP Therapeutic Stance

ERP is a brief procedure, during which the therapist maintains an emphatic and confident position that resonates with the truth that *that* event is in the past and the patient is in the present. When using ERP, the therapist's stance should be the same described by Dr. Francine Shapiro (2001) for working with a patient during an abreaction:

> *The clinician should maintain a position of detached compassion in relation to the patient.* (p. 174)

She goes on to say:

> *To increase the patient's sense of safety, follow the "golden rule" of "Do unto others . . ." That is, the clinician should ask himself/herself what kind of support he would want if he were suddenly flooded with the emotions and physical sensations of childhood terror. The answer will probably reveal the importance of something that conveys an atmosphere of nurturing and trust and makes the clinician feel that it is safe to proceed. On the basis of this assumption, the patient should be continually reassured that the clinician is calm, caring, unsurprised by the content of the abreaction, supportive of its manifestations (regardless of how intensely expressed), and responsible for the safety of the situation.* (p. 175)

The fully present clinician and his recurrent supportive words have a strong grounding effect on patients after critical incidents. This results in patients reorienting back into the present time. The clinician's words, eye contact, and BLS are added elements that serve to anchor patients more solidly within that present time and safer location.

History-Taking

Patients who benefit from ERP are those who have difficulty telling a coherent history; patients in a state of silent terror cannot say anything at first while those in a highly agitated state have difficulty in telling very much history. If a patient cannot communicate, information about the incident is reported to the clinician by the ambulance or hospital staff. A more complete history regarding the immediate trauma can be done after the patient becomes verbal, once the ERP has been effective at establishing a present orientation (that the patient is safe from the recent dangerous event).

Assessment

In the Standard EMDR Protocol, the Assessment Phase allows patients to fully access their memory of the event on all levels. In the highly agitated state of Acute Stress Reaction (ASR), patients are very much in their internal world, already actively accessing the memory fully on the sensory, emotional, and body levels. Therefore, the formal Assessment Phase of EMDR is not necessary and the informal assessment proceeds as follows:

- The assumed initial negative cognition (NC): "I am in danger," or "My family or friends are in danger."
- The assumed initial positive cognition (PC): "I am/they are safe now from that event."
- The term *from that event* is added to give truth to the PC, allowing for ongoing danger (e.g., war, terrorism, natural disaster).
- Emotion is assumed to be high fear or terror.
- Subjective Units of Disturbance (SUD) is assumed to be at or close to 7–10 +, where 0 is no disturbance and 10 is the worst disturbance imaginable.
- Body sensation: The therapist observes the body sensations such as muscle tension, catatonia, shaking uncontrollably, breathing rapidly, and so forth.

EMDR and Positive Cognitions

In using positive cognitions in the face of critical incidents, this author learned that saying, "You are safe now," was not sufficient to help patients return to the present. "No, I am not safe; the missiles are still landing and the bombs are still exploding," was their frequent retort. When adding, however, the words, ". . . from the past event" (as in "You are safe now, from the past event"), patients were able to calm down, reorient, and view this statement as a true positive cognition. The adding of, "It is over," reinforced, "You are safe now from that past event." A felt sense of present safety from that past event was highly instrumental in helping them to cope with/manage future events during which they could again be in danger.

Bilateral Stimulation (BLS)

The bilateral stimulation (BLS) used during the Desensitization Phase of ERP is based on the EMDR concept of utilizing dual attention. A patient is already accessing the past event as if it is happening now (first attention) and this is the cause of the distress. The patient, in the current reality of being in the emergency room (ER), is now safe (second attention) from the recent traumatic event. BLS is used in conjunction with the phrase, *"You are safe now from that past event."*

- *Type of BLS:* Since tapping does not require active cooperation, it is used throughout the ERP processing.
- *Speed of BLS:* Bilateral stimulation is offered at a rate as fast as the patient can follow or at a variable speed to keep patients in the present. Although in EMDR, patients may close their eyes when using tapping, it is most often helpful when using ERP to keep eyes open to secure a present orientation. After patients again become verbal or can begin to follow instructions, tapping accompanied by having them observe (the bilateral tapping) can be a powerful combination. It should be noted that patients who follow the tapping with their eyes will often be unable to keep up with the higher speed used when one BLS modality is used alone. The speed should thus be reduced to allow the patient to follow.

Sound (auditory) BLS is not often utilized as noise can trigger an aspect of the recent dangerous situation such as the sound of a missile landing or a crash. If eye movements or tapping are not available or useful, sound BLS can cautiously (and quietly) be attempted.

Ending Goals for ERP Patients

Patients who were initially verbal will be able to express their recognition of current safety and will demonstrate body language reflecting increased calm. Most patients will still have a degree of agitation. This can be seen as ecological for their current state. The goals of ERP are reached when patients exhibit:

- Recognition of being in the present
- Recovery of the ability to communicate verbally
- Demonstration of body language suggesting a calmer state
- Ability to respond to the SUDs scale (SUDs = 3–5/10)

Moving Beyond Safety Concerns Into Responsibility Concerns

There are situations where establishing that a particular danger is in the past and that safety is in place will not be sufficient to bring down disturbance levels to a large degree below 3–5/10. At this stage, the patient is no longer in the "speechless terror" state (which may have been resolved by the ERP establishing current safety from that past event). Here, clients are most often verbal but can still be highly agitated. This often happens when there is a feeling of responsibility or lack of control and choices (i.e., following failed rescue attempts). In such cases, a focus on safety may not reduce distress during a desensitization or installation.

The script below, under "Addressing Responsibility Concerns," may present a viable option to try when no progress has been made using safety as the target and when the patient is verbal and making comments such as "I should have done something," "I did something wrong," or "It's my fault."

Closure and Follow Up

This is a good time to ask for permission to contact patients at a later date to see how they are doing. In cases of emergency intervention with ongoing danger, a face-to-face follow-up session may not easily occur. However, at this point, the patient is verbal and you can request a phone number along with a friend or relative's phone number, and ask permission to contact them at an approximate time interval (week, month, etc.). Most patients are grateful and offer a positive response. Since you may not be able to contact them during times of ongoing danger, it is important not to say you *will*, but instead, you *may* call them.

According to the protocols of the emergency room, a patient is given a final medical exam before being released. In addition, the patient is given a fact sheet describing common physiological and emotional symptoms occurring within the first 48 to 72 hours of involvement in a traumatic incident. Examples may include flashbacks, difficulty sleeping, and increased sensitivity to loud noises. Also listed are unusually strong reactions such as increased anger and withdrawal. It is mentioned that most patients will usually experience steady improvement over the following month. Referral numbers are listed should further psychological treatment be desired.

Training and ERP

This procedure presumes clinician familiarity with the Standard EMDR Protocol from which it is adapted. Clinicians highly experienced in dealing with patients immediately after a traumatic event—who are not familiar with EMDR—may still benefit from this protocol.

Note: The ERP procedure has not received official sanction or endorsement from the EMDR Institute; however, it is in the early stages of being empirically investigated. To date, clinician and patient anecdotal reports are encouraging with an informal study (small N) by the author, suggesting that 75% of the patients who received treatment as usual (ie, no ERP) presented with PTSD two years post-trauma, compared to 25% who receiving ERP.

Emergency Response Procedure and Script

Phase 1: History Taking

Introduce yourself to the patient.

> Say, *"I am _____ (state your name). What happened to you that brought you here now?"*

_____

_____

_____

Note: Usually this will be a brief report of what they have experienced if they are verbal. It helps establish a level of rapport and connection to the present. For those patients who do not respond, move to Phase 2: Preparation.

Phase 2: Preparation

Initial Preparation

If the patient is shaking uncontrollably or feeling overwhelmed, it is essential to normalize this behavior.

Say, *"Your current shaking, rapid heartbeat, and breathing _____ (or whatever signs the patient is showing) is the body's normal healthy way of dealing with a dangerous situation."*

Preparation

Give a brief explanation describing EMDR.

Say, *"I will be using a procedure based on what your body and mind do naturally to deal with strong emotional experiences, which is similar to the natural state of dreaming when your eyes move rapidly back and forth. This can
help you learn new things and be calm. It will also help you come back to the
present. I am going to ask you to follow my fingers with your eyes, or with
your permission, I am going to tap on your hands. If you would like me to
stop, just raise your hand. Would that be okay with you?"*

If the patient does not respond add the following:

Say, *"I understand that you are extremely preoccupied with this event you have
been through and are not talking now. I will assume you agree to do this
procedure unless you say no or shake your head no."*

If there is any possibility of neck injury, do not ask them to shake their heads.

Phase 3: Assessment

The formal Assessment Phase of EMDR is *not* necessary and the informal assessment proceeds assuming the following: negative cognition (NC) = "I am in danger," or "My family or friends are in danger"; initial positive cognition (PC) = "I am/they are safe now *from that event*"; emotion = high fear or terror; Subjective Units of Disturbance = 7–10+ /10 (worst); body sensation = therapist's observation of patient's body sensations such as muscle tension, catatonia, shaking uncontrollably, breathing rapidly, and so forth.

Phase 4: Desensitization

Introduce Dual Attention and BLS

The way to use dual attention is by repeating the following:

Say, *"You are in the ER and safe now from that past event. That is over."*

In the case where the safety of family members is not known, say the following:

Say, *"That event is over. What has happened is over and in the past."*

Patients are directed to focus on the here and now of being safe in the hospital (or wherever they currently are) and away from the flashbacks of the incident despite their shaking bodies.

Say, *"You are in the hospital* (or wherever they are) *now and are safe from that
past event. That is over."*

If there are flashbacks of the incident, use BLS (such as eye movements or hand tapping) together with the therapist's voice, and bring the patient back to the present and current reality of safety. See below.

Begin BLS. At first, there can be a re-experiencing of trauma followed by calming and the ability to communicate.

Say, *"I am going to ask you to follow my fingers with your eyes or, with your
permission, I am going to tap on your hands."*

Note: In the event a patient has a problem with the clinician touching her, a pen or any other neutral object can be used for light tapping.

Begin BLS.

> Say, *"You are in the emergency room* (or wherever the patient is) *and you are safe. That event is over out there. You are safe here in the emergency room (or wherever the patient is). Focus on being in the* _____ (place the patient is presently located) *and safe, notice my being with you, listen to my voice, and feel my hands tapping on yours (or notice my hands moving)."*

Do BLS. Repeat the above statements during each set (as during abreaction) or approximately every 5 to 10 sets. BLS can be given in short or long sets or with varying speed during a set as is done during abreaction in EMDR. Stopping points can be when the patient appears to relax somewhat or starts to be verbal. Otherwise, a traditional set of 24 can be used.

> Say, *"Take a breath. Let it go. What are you noticing?"*

_____

_____

If a patient does not verbally respond, say the following:

> Say, *"Just notice what is happening,"* while doing more BLS and repeating the statement, *"You are safe now from that event that is over and you are in the* _____ (place where the person is located)."

Continue this until you see the patient's body calming and the patient is able to tell you what she is noticing.

> Say, *"Take a breath. Let it go. What are you noticing?"*

_____

_____

For patients who present in a state of silent terror and are nonverbal, being able to communicate and recognize current safety can be seen as a stopping place. A completed SUD, in this situation, would be approximately 3–5/10, as inferred from body language or expressed by the patient.

Optional:

Note: In ERP, do not ask the patient to, "think of the incident."

> Say *"On a scale from 0 to 10, where 0 is no disturbance or neutral and 10 is the highest disturbance you can imagine, how disturbing does it feel now?"*

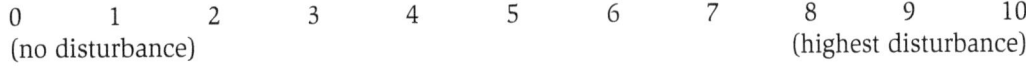

0   1   2   3   4   5   6   7   8   9   10
(no disturbance)   (highest disturbance)

Phase 5: Installation

Formal EMDR installation is not done. Instead, assess the patient's awareness of current safety and location.

> Say, *"Where are you now?"*

_____

_____

When patients state the experience of being oriented and currently safe in the ER (or wherever they are), say the following:

Say, *"Are you able to recognize that you are currently safe and that the past, dangerous event is over?"*

_____

_____

When present safety recognition is not sufficient to allow closure, the difficulty may be a sense of lack of control/choice. If the patient says: *"But it's still dangerous and another attack/missile landing/earthquake can happen when I leave here,"* say the following:

Say, *"Yes, in the future there are many different things that can happen but what we have found is that letting yourself be in the present—here right now—can be helpful to figure out how to deal with those later situations even if it is 5 minutes from now. Can you let yourself realize that at this moment you are here and safe now with me? Because you are safe, right now. What happened is over. And later we can try to figure out a way to make sure you remain as safe as is possible, but now just notice that right now you are here and you are safe. All these other things can be dealt with much more easily when you can let yourself just be here safe right now."*

Note: Receiving a patient's engaged, affirmative response to the question regarding whether she can now recognize that she is safe is critical. That affirmation indicates that the patient has been able to reorient not only to "place" but also to "time." This means that the patient is aware that she is beyond the past threat/danger.

Sometimes a person needs to be reminded of real life solutions:

Say, *"What have you been told to do by the police if another siren goes off and you are in the car to keep you reasonably safe?"*

_____

_____

Say, *"Go with that."* Do BLS.

Once this has been accomplished, do not return the focus to the original incident. Instead, proceed to closure.

Addressing Responsibility Concerns (as Needed)

Should the client express comments that reflect self-blame, or a shift to the domain of responsibility, you can attempt to ask a clarifying question:

Say, *"Is there more about what just happened that you wish to tell me that can help us understand what may be keeping the distress from getting less? Feel free to tell me just what you are comfortable telling me now."*

_____

_____

Within the time frame that ERP treatment allows, it is very difficult to find a true, positive cognition when dealing with issues of responsibility. Therefore, after acknowledging the issue of responsibility, it is deferred for now. It will be dealt with by EMD or R-TEP (see below) or at a different time. In ERP we then return to "You are here now and that event is over" as a first step in the direction of dealing with any of the other issues or actions they may need to do later.

Say, "At times like this, it is common to try to find someone responsible for this terrible incident. You might blame yourself or blame others. But right now, whatever the reason that this happened, even though it is a horrible thing that happened, what has happened has occurred in the past and you are here right now. Being able to just let yourself know that you are here now and that this event is over is an important step for what needs to be done next. So please allow my tapping/hand movement to help you realize that you are here now—for whatever reason it happened—and you can be here this moment. Recognizing you are here now can help you deal with the other things you will need to do later. If this issue remains it can be addressed at a later time."

At this point, most clients are at a reduced level of distress and you can move on to Closure.

Note: If the client still remains distressed, she may wish to talk more about the traumatic incident. If time permits, the following is recommended.

Narrative of Event

At this point, it is possible for patients to give a narrative of what they experienced. Do not push for details. This narrative is therapeutic. This can be helpful as it is using left-brain processing to establish the proper sense of past, present, and future.

Say, "Please tell me what happened from just prior to the start of the event until now. Feel free to tell me just what you are comfortable relating."

_____
_____
_____
_____
_____
_____

Very often, in telling the narrative, the client may remember details, temporarily forgotten, that could free them of a sense of responsibility. Or, they realize that they were more active than they remembered and therefore have a better sense of control than they originally thought. At other times, this narrative reveals another cognition that is an additional source of stress, such as a false sense of responsibility as in survival guilt, as mentioned above. Common negative cognitions are "I should have done something," or, "I did something wrong" (by not warning others or not saving other victims). In this case, EMD or R-TEP (Shapiro & Laub, 2009) may be utilized, if time permits. This may not be possible during mass trauma as many people are in need of immediate treatment.

If patients have not been able to calm down using ERP, other standard non-EMDR types of treatment such as medication can be utilized.

Phase 6: Body Scan

Body Scan is not formally done but the ability to verbalize, cessation of shaking, and noticeable calming of the body will indicate an ability to move to closure. It can be seen as normal for many people to be agitated up to two to three days following a traumatic incident.

Phase 7: Closure

Closure is done stating the following:

Say, "It is common to have a reaction to what has happened to you. You might have flashbacks of what happened, difficulty sleeping, and a number of emotions such as distress, fear, or anger. You may notice that you are much more jumpy and startle more easily by loud sounds or anything that reminds you of what happened. If you find these symptoms lasting longer than 2 to 3 days and not subsiding, this is not unusual, but we can help you to handle these reactions so that you will be calmer. Here are some numbers to call (give contact information), *if you would like more assistance. Do you have any questions?"*

_____

_____

If follow up is indicated, ask permission to contact them at a later date to see how they are doing.

Say, *"Would it be ok for you to give me your phone number and a family or friend's phone number so that I may call to follow up and find out how you are?"*

_____

_____

Say, *"I will try to follow up, but, if I can't, or if you need more assistance, please don't hesitate to call the numbers on the sheet for further help."*

Phase 8: Reevaluation

If you do have the opportunity for a follow up meeting, it is helpful to administer an Impact of Events scale to help assess if the patient needs further treatment and for use in research.

Acknowledgments

I would like to acknowledge Debby Zucker, EMDR Consultant, Clinical Social Worker, and Medic, who has utilized ERP during her emergency work with patients in ambulances. I would also like to thank Karen Lansing, LMFT, BCETS, Rosalie Thomas, PhD, and John Reiman, PhD, in the development of this chapter.

Most of all, I would like to thank Marilyn Luber, PhD, who tirelessly worked with me. Her vast knowledge as an EMDR expert and her ability to ask those perfect, insightful, and revealing questions, enabled me to discover and then articulate the elements that may be responsible for ERP's effectiveness.

SUMMARY SHEET:
Emergency Response Procedure (ERP)

1A

Gary Quinn
SUMMARY SHEET BY MARILYN LUBER

Name:_____ Diagnosis:_____
Medications: _____

☑ Check when task is completed or response has changed or to indicate symptoms.

Note: This material is meant as a checklist for your response. Please keep in mind that it is only a reminder of different tasks that may or may not apply to your incident.

Phase 1: History Taking

History by Patient: _____ History from Hospital Staff: _____

_____
_____
_____
_____
_____
_____
_____
_____
_____
_____
_____
_____
_____

Phase 2: Preparation

Physical Symptoms: _____
_____

Explanation of ERP	☐ Completed _____	Time
Agreement to do ERP	☐ Completed _____	Time

Phase 3: Assessment

Assumed NC: "I am in danger."
Assumed PC: "I am safe NOW *from that event*."
Emotion: High fear or terror
SUD: 10/10
Body Sensation: (Therapist observation) _____

_____

Introduce Dual Attention and BLS: ☐ Completed _____ Time

Phase 4: Desensitization

Therapist: *"You are in the emergency room* (or wherever they are) *and you are safe. That event is over out there. You are safe here in the emergency room. Focus on being in the hospital and safe, notice my standing with you, listen to my voice, and feel my hands tapping on yours."*

Stop when patient appears to relax somewhat or starts to be verbal.

Note patient response: When patient who was in silent terror/nonverbal, exhibits shifts in body posture, can communicate and recognizes current safety with SUD around 3–5/10, this is a stopping place.

Change in body posture:	☐ Completed	_____ Time
Starting to communicate:	☐ Completed	_____ Time
Recognize current safety:	☐ Completed	_____ Time
Degree of agitation SUD:	_____/10	

Phase 5: Installation (Formal Installation Not Done)

Oriented to location:	☐ Completed	_____ Time
Recognition currently safe:	☐ Completed	_____ Time
Recognition event is over:	☐ Completed	_____ Time

If patient still feels threatened: Say, *"And yes, in the future there are many different things that can happen but what we have found is that letting yourself be in the present—here right now—can be helpful to figure out how to deal with those later situations even if it is 5 minutes from now. Can you let yourself realize that at this moment you are here and safe now with me? Because you are safe, right now. What happened is over. And later we can try to figure out a way to make sure you remain as safe as is possible, but now just notice that right now you are here and you are safe. All these other things can be dealt with much more easily when you can let yourself just be here safe right now."* ☐ Completed _____ Time

Responsibility concerns (as needed): Say, *"At times like this, it is common to try to find someone responsible for this terrible incident. You might blame yourself or blame others. But right now, whatever the reason that this happened, even though it is horrible, what has occurred is in the past and you are here right now. Being able to just let yourself know that you are here now and that this event is over is an important step for what needs to be done next. So, please allow my tapping/hand movement to help you realize that you are here now—for whatever reason it happened—and you can be here this moment. Recognizing you are here now can help you deal with the other things you will need to do later. If this issue remains, it can be addressed at a later time."*

Summary Sheet: Emergency Response Procedure (ERP)   15

Narrative of Event (Optional) : Use EMD or R-TEP, if time permits.

_____
_____
_____
_____
_____
_____
_____
_____
_____
_____

Target/Memory/Image: _____
_____

PC: _____
VoC: _____/7
NC: _____
Emotions: _____
SUD: _____/10
Sensation: _____

Phase 6: Body Scan (Formal Body Scan Not Done)

Can verbalize calming of body: ☐ Completed _____ Time

Phase 7: Closure

Therapist: "*It is common to have a reaction to what has happened to you. You might have flashbacks of what happened, difficulty sleeping, and a number of emotions such as distress, fear, or anger. You may notice that you are much more jumpy and startle more easily by loud sounds or anything that reminds you of what happened. If you find these symptoms lasting longer than 2 to 3 days and not subsiding, this is not unusual but we can help you to handle these reactions so that you will be calmer. Here are some numbers to call _____ [give contact information), if you would like more assistance. Do you have any questions?*"

Medical evaluation: ☐ Completed _____ Time
Given fact sheet on common symptoms: ☐ Completed _____ Time
Referral numbers as needed: ☐ Completed _____ Time

Phase 8: Reevaluation

Contact within the week: ☐ Completed _____ Date

EMDR Emergency Room and Wards Protocol (EMDR-ER©)

Judith S. B. Guedalia and Frances R. Yoeli

Introduction

The EMDR-Emergency Room and Wards Protocol (EMDR-ER©) was developed by Dr. Judith Guedalia, after being present at more than 26 Mass Casualty Events (MCEs). She and the other members of Shaare Zedek Medical Center's Trauma Team attended to more than 38% of the 1,623 patients injured in Jerusalem terror attacks during the "Second Intifada." The Second Intifada spanned nearly 4 years, lasting from November 2000 until September 2004.

EMDR Emergency Room and Wards Protocol (EMDR-ER) Script

Phase 1: History Taking

Screening

The EMDR-ER Protocol is used with patients who do not seem able to move on to the ambulatory staging area (i.e., are still on gurneys, frozen on a chair, or on a hospital bed), and who display difficulty in being able to reassume normal appropriate affect, physical, psychological, or behavioral functions at an adequate level given the situation.

Since patients are usually in the emergency room (ER) for many, many hours (5 to 8 hours), there are numerous opportunities to assess the patient's ability to communicate by various means, including just being nearby, standing, or sitting next to the patient—whether the patient is on a chair, gurney, bed, and so forth, or doing a more formal type of assessment. Once the patient reaches a basic level of safety, the therapist then can begin communicating safety phrases to the patient. The criteria for the patient reaching a basic level of safety are the following: shows a basic level of physical relatedness, can focus eyes, can respond to questions, looks around the gurney or chair, shows interest at some level of the surroundings, and breathing cadence slows down to normal.

When the patient shows a basic level of safety, the therapist can nod, hold the patient's hand, and breathe in the same cadence as the patient. At this point of the patient's recovery, it is not necessary to respond to questions asked by the patient with verbal answers. This is because verbal areas of the brain may have shut down and the acutely stressed patient may not hear answers but can sense presence and holding. Very often, patients in this situation have not been able to relate to language, as evidenced by repeating the same questions despite the answers given. Often, they are in a dissociative-like state that is more of a biological response to acute stress. This state need not be labelled or medicated immediately.

The next step is for the therapist to begin to say short, comforting, and grounding phrases such as the following:

"You are alive";
"You are safe now";
"You are in the hospital";
"I am here for you."

When this level of trust and safety is achieved, the work begins to move forward. Installing a sense of safety, trust, and the realization that they are among the living, is facilitated by the presence of a trained EMDR clinician. Once the sense of immediate safety is established, the introduction of the EMDR-ER protocol is possible and recommended. This protocol can be used with good results even with patients who speak a different language than the therapist; however, an interpreter might be helpful.

When the patient is showing dissociative responses to the trauma such as hysterical paralysis or a fugue-like state, do not attempt any EMDR. Also, EMDR is not used in the ER with patients who seem to have below borderline intelligence, as assessed by clinically administered (bedside) tests such as the Mini Mental State Examination (MMSE). The needs of these patients are different. Repetition in a quiet environment—without a lot of stimulation of the ER—may be better for them. EMDR may be too stimulating for them.

Receiving permission to engage the patient in some form of bilateral stimulation (BLS) is frequently not possible during the initial stages of hospitalization. When a patient cannot provide permission—and BLS might still be appropriate—only a physician or nurse is allowed to touch the patient. Once the clinician has received an okay to touch the patient from the patient himself, BLS in the form of tapping is possible.

Phase 2: Preparation

Safe Contact—With Dual Attention Elements

The patients are generally prone on a gurney (possibly compounding the drawing of attention inward to their recent trauma). With medical permission, check if the patient can be raised or somewhat raised to a sitting position and then say the following:

Say, *"Hello, my name is _____ (state name)."*

Then say, *"You are in the hospital now and you are safe. Is it okay for me to touch you here?"*

_____

_____

If the client nods his head, it is taken as an agreement that permits touch. If the patient does not agree, go into the cognitive explanation before conducting bilateral stimulation with touch.

Point to where you will touch the patient.

With those who cannot respond verbally at this time, either touch in two places, or stand in their line of vision as well as touching them. This draws their attention outward to the safe present; this is the ER type of "Dual Attention" that keeps the patient in the *present* and provides a reality check to the fact that they are now *safe*. The external attention created by the touch, the calm tone of voice, and the safe presence of the therapist in the patient's line of vision is particularly important for the hyper-aroused patient who requires grounding.

Introduce the EMDR-ER Protocol or Intervention With a Cognitive Neuropsychological Lesson

> Say, *"When we experience trauma, our brain takes in many sounds, feelings, images, smells, and even tastes, all at the same time. This avalanche of sensations coupled with the very real fear of dying, gets encoded or locked in our brain. The area of the brain that is generally activated in such situations is called the limbic system. This is the area that stores and processes emotion in our brain. This area experiences memories and is not generally seen as accessible by speech."*

We use this further explanation to encourage the patient's recovery and cooperation.

> Say, *"This is especially true soon after the event has occurred* (this seems to be a neuropsychological reality). *Initially trauma is a cortical experience in the limbic system, specifically the hippocampus. The hippocampus is an area of the brain that looks like a seahorse. It is responsible for episodic memory and spatial navigation. Unlike motor memory such as remembering how to ride a bicycle or swim, or factual memory such as recalling dates of historical events, episodic memory involves day-to-day, short-term memories—what we did yesterday, or whom we met last week. It is the area that scientists now understand to be affected in traumatic experiences. What seems to occur is very visceral* (internal in the brain) *and is not neuropsychologically available for verbal encoding. The senses such as feeling, seeing, smelling, hearing, and taste are the modalities by which information is received, processed, and encoded by the brain. Research has shown* (and our clinical experience has found) *that before these images, smells, sounds, and so forth get stored, it is beneficial to talk and give words to these sensory inputs so as to allow them to be available for verbal access in the future."*

This may be very complicated and wordy for the ER patient. But the presence of the therapist's voice and the explanation, well understood or not, tends to foster a sense of calm and safety. In general, we begin this after the patient is somewhat stabilized. Also, it gives family members something to hang onto once we begin. They may be afraid of responses that we understand to be normal for Acute Stress Disorder (ASD) patients. Also, some aspects of the cognitive intervention may be understood and begin to help the patient formulate a frame of reference and then build on it in a logical scaffolding sort of way.

Phase 3: Assessment

It is important for the therapist to be there with acceptance and the safety of her physical presence. This seems to act as an affirmation of the patient's existence. The clinician's presence creates a dual attention; the therapist assists the patient to move from an internal focus to an external focus as he is now safe and becomes more aware of that safety in the present with the therapist. You might whisper, again to reinforce the reality of the situation.

> Say, *"You are alive," "You are safe now,"* or *"You did get away from there."*

Listen to the Patient's Narrative or Story of the Event

Attend to body language during the recitation of the story. Note if there is agitation in the patient's vocabulary that is specific to individual or cultural background punctuating the narrative, for example, "Time stopped," "I can't move (speak or hear)," or "I am dead," and use this to reflect or suggest negative cognitions (NCs) such as "I am helpless," "I am out of control," or "I am going to die (am dying)." Take notes without interrupting or asking for clarification.

> Say, *"Please tell me what happened."*

_____

_____

___

Target, Memory, or Image of the Actual Traumatic Event

Say, *"Please allow yourself to focus on an image, picture, or sound of the event."*

___

Image

Say, *"What do you see now?"*

___

Positive Cognition (PC)

The NC and PC are reversed in order to further affirm, enforce, enhance, and embed the issues of safety, control, and recovery. It is TOO early for the patient to say, "I am in control" or that "I will be ok"; safe and alive are the most positive we can get.

Say, *"When you bring up that image, can you now feel that you are alive and safe?"*

___

Note: Some humor may be appropriate here.

Say, *"I am alive and speaking to you, which proves to me that you are also alive."*

Clinical experience has demonstrated that when patients respond with a smile, it is diagnostic and tells us that they have available resources. They may not truly believe that they *are* alive and that they survived the incident.

Validity of Cognition (VoC)

Say, *"When you think of the incident* (or picture), *how true do those words _____ (clinician repeats the positive cognition) feel to you now on a scale of 1 to 7, where 1 feels completely false and 7 feels completely true?"*

1	2	3	4	5	6	7
(completely false)						(completely true)

Negative Cognition (NC)

Say, *"What words go best with that picture and expresses your negative thinking and belief about yourself now?"*

_____

_____

_____

Emotions

Say, *"When you bring up that picture or incident and those words (repeat the NC), what emotion(s) do you feel now?"*

_____

_____

_____

Note: Connect the patient's words to the emotion in order to narrow the distance between the words and feelings or the cognitive and the visceral. Don't be afraid to show your own emotions—by crying or sighing—as it can help the patient emote and expresses your own genuineness and empathy.

Subjective Units of Disturbance (SUD)

Say, *"On a scale of 0 to 10, where 0 is no disturbance or neutral and 10 is the highest disturbance you can imagine, how disturbing does it feel now?"*

0	1	2	3	4	5	6	7	8	9	10
(no disturbance)										(highest disturbance)

Note: This question can evoke an abreaction and therefore it is not necessary to insist on a SUD at this point.

Location of Body Sensation

Say, *"Where do you feel it in your body?"*

_____

_____

Note: This question can be problematic when the patients are physically injured. In such cases, this question should not be asked.

Phase 4: Desensitization

Ask the patient to repeat the narrative and pay close attention to what the patient is saying and to your notes from previous visits to this patient. Be aware of what can be used from the narrative as a metaphor that can distance them from the scene such as video, reversed binoculars, television, or other nonreminders of the situation that brought him to the ER. Be attuned to the use of words in the past tense, "I saw," "The sounds were," "He was," and so forth, as opposed to using the present tense.

> Say, *"Please tell me again what happened. Sometimes, it is helpful to think about it as if it were on television or that you are looking at it with reversed binoculars* (or any other relevant metaphors).*"*

_____
_____
_____
_____
_____

As time in the ER goes on, and the patients are off the gurneys and onto chairs, it is sometimes feasible to do bilateral stimulation (BLS). However, there is usually no private space that is quiet or secluded enough to comfortably carry this out. Subtle tapping on hands, shoulders, or knees may be more suitable as active cooperation is not required here.

> Say, *"I am going to touch you gently on your* _____ (hands, shoulders, knees—wherever is appropriate or accessible); *this may help you to feel more comfortable."*

In a Mass Casualty Event (MCE), there is generally a low patient-to-staff ratio (more injured than available staff members). This may be particularly true of the psychology and social work staff members, as each patient may bring twice as many family members in need of assistance and guidance. With this fact in mind, the therapist keeps going around and coming back to each patient. Using notes to keep track of what time the therapist was last with the client is helpful, as well as the specifics and sequence of the patient's narrative. During some MCEs, there may be tens of patients per therapist.

The therapist continues to return to the patient and restarts the processing. The time lapses tend to reduce or dilute the emotion of the narrative (a form of titration) and this reinforces the processing. When the therapist leaves to move on to someone else, she gives him homework, such as breathing exercises, if this is not physically painful. It is important to keep reinforcing that the patient is in the hospital and is in a safe place now.

> Say, *"Please tell me again what happened. Sometimes, it is helpful to think about it as if it were on television or that you are looking at it with reversed binoculars* (or any other relevant metaphor).*"*

_____
_____
_____
_____
_____

> Say, *"Okay. I want to tell you that you are safe now. You are in the hospital and you are safe here with us. I will be back soon. While I am gone, please focus on something that you can see right here and then count your breaths—each inhale and each exhale—in your mind with your mouth closed. If there is another breathing exercise you like to do, go ahead and do that."*

This tends to keep the patient (and family members) busy and less focused on his traumatic experience, literally externalizing his energies.

Each time the therapist returns to the specific patient, she refocuses the patient by being in his line of vision or touching him on his arm or other noninjured area. The therapist speaks softly if his eyes are closed. Generally, the patient does NOT want to close his eyes, as the images that he sees then are so horrific, he prefers to leave his eyes open. The therapist might suggest that he close his eyes once assuring him that she is standing near, thereby reinforcing the safe place.

Say, *"If it is helpful, you might want to close your eyes now knowing that I am right here with you and you are safe now in the hospital."*

Phase 5: Installation

The therapist uses her notes from the last time she saw the patient as a scaffold to build a richer, more complete story. Generally the therapist might emphasize or reframe any reference to acts of kindness or positive experiences the patient referred to in his narrative. Repeat the narrative again, interweaving new information and the positive experience, checking the patient's physical and emotional state while using BLS if possible.

Help incorporate sequences such as time and place concepts into a narrative.

"What time did you leave the house, office, or school?"
"What happened next…?"
"Where were you standing, sitting, or walking?"

Say, *" _____ (repeat the narrative building in a more complete story)."*

As the therapist repeats the story, it is important to utilize the patient's own words, where possible. The idea is to amplify the points made and help him understand the sequence of his narrative so that he has a cohesive experience of what happened to him and gains a sense of control, self-determination, power, and a sense that it is "worth it" to continue living, notwithstanding what has just happened and that he will be released from the safe hospital space. The narrative that is created will be the one that will (hopefully) be crystallized for future reference. This process may take hours! Continue repeating the narrative above as needed.

Emotions

Say, *"When you bring up that picture or incident, and those words _____ (repeat the PC), what emotion(s) do you feel now?"*

_____

_____

_____

Note: Connect his words to the emotion in order to narrow the distance between the words and feelings or the cognitive and the visceral. Again, don't be afraid to show your own emotions—by crying or sighing—as it can help the patient emote and expresses your own genuineness and empathy.

Subjective Units of Disturbance (SUD)

Say, *"On a scale of 0 to 10, where 0 is no disturbance or neutral and 10 is the highest disturbance you can imagine, how disturbing does it feel now?"*

0   1   2   3   4   5   6   7   8   9   10
(no disturbance)   (highest disturbance)

Note: This question can evoke an abreaction and therefore it is not necessary to insist on a SUD at this point.

Location of Body Sensation

Say, *"Where do you feel it in your body?"*

_____

_____

Note: This question can be problematic when the patients are physically injured. In such cases, this question should not be asked.

Do this until the patient has reprocessed the event and demonstrated that he is "speech-full," that is, the patient is able to give at least some words to verbalize the sensory experiences, or a coherent account with generally appropriate affect.

Reduction of Observable SUD

The goal is to get the patient up and out of the gurney, chair, bed, and the ER, on their way home through the exit processes. This means that the therapist probably will not get the target to go down to a SUD of 0; however, the patient's physical movement off of the existing ER place (gurney, bed, or chair) is viewed as a decrease in the SUD.

Phase 6: Body Scan

In the ER, when using the EMDR-ER Intervention/Protocol, attention to the body is directed at checking differences and changes in the patient's emotional tone such as in the following: stopping uncontrollable crying, more control of emotional reactions, and the decrease of physical signs such as uncontrollable shaking, perspiring, and perseverative verbalizations.

As the process goes on, rather than specifically asking the patient for a Body Scan, which, with the physically injured, tends to have another connotation (the patient may give a more medical symptom review rather than a measure of tensions still affecting the body), the therapist watches for changes in body language such as slower cadence of speech and fuller breathing. Also, other more verbal signs of change may be the following: a richness fills out the narrative, and the patient begins worrying about specifics such as "Where is my wallet?" "How will I get home?" "My passport or ID is missing." Another good sign (of return to normal rather than hyperarousal and in-trauma functioning) is when the patient starts to say "I'm hungry."

The Body Scan is more appropriate at the final discharge staging area, when the primary purpose is to check for residual, unprocessed information that is thought to be stored as sensory or body memories, and may require further processing so as to further reduce tension and lead into closure at a future time. This information should be relayed to the patient and his family as part of the cognitive discharge process (immediately before or after the medical discharge process—see the following).

Phase 7: Closure

Final Feedback

Final feedback occurs when the patient repeats the narrative in the presence of the internist or physician and in the presence of a social worker, psychologist, or psychiatrist. This takes place during the final medical check that ascertains that the patient has had all the tests: x-rays, blood tests, medical specialist evaluations, and so forth, which were initially ordered in the ER. The patient's delivery of the narrative is assessed and when it is deemed cohesive and affect is appropriate, the patient is released from the trauma (MCE) process.

Say, *"Please tell us about what happened to you."*

_____
_____

The patient receives a prepared handout with information concerning the normal responses that may occur to someone after being present during, for example, an explosion that may cause ringing ears, acute stress, sleep disruptions, and nightmares, and the telephone numbers to call for further treatment (outpatient clinic). This, then, is the final medical exam and the patient is seen by a social worker, psychiatrist, or psychologist before being discharged.

Say, *"Here is a handout that tells you about what to expect after an event such as what happened to you. It also gives you the telephone numbers that you can call for further help or treatment. You may still have a day or two of disrupted sleep, you might find yourself startling more often, or you may have other signs of stress. I want you to know that this is normal in light of the terrible experience that you have been through. If you find that these symptoms are lasting longer than a few days and do not seem to be subsiding, be sure to ask for further help by calling someone who is listed on this sheet. If for some reason you cannot find your sheet, you can always telephone us or come back here and someone here can give you the information that you need. Do you have any questions?"*

_____
_____

Social Services Consultation and Release

This can be tailored to your circumstances. In this situation, the social worker verifies that there is a home to go to, and that the person is not a tourist who will be alone in a hotel, and that there is someone to pick up the individual from the ER. The patient is then given an official release form from the hospital, along with the phone number of Bituach Leumi (Israeli National Insurance), and the code number of this specific MCE for future reference (all of this is printed out and handed to the patient).

Say, *"Where will you go when you leave here?"*

_____
_____

Say, *"Do you have someone to pick you up now?"*

_____
_____

Say, *"Here is your official release from the hospital _____ (and any other information that needs to be given)."*

Phase 8: Reevaluation

This phase can be tailored to your needs. In this situation, patients are generally required to come back for follow up of their medical conditions within a day or two; others who are not as physically injured are told to get in contact with their family physician and Bituach Leumi if they don't live near the hospital and can call our Post-MCE/Trauma/Acute Stress Psycho-Social Department. Within a few days, the national insurance agency arranges a phone call by an assigned social worker who will become the case manager for this patient. As a result of research and clinical experience throughout Israel, patients are eligible for group therapy or other services as deemed necessary by the agency in charge of the MCE/Terror victims once the event has been classified as such.

SUMMARY SHEET: EMDR Emergency Room and Wards Protocol (EMDR-ER©)

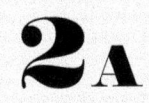

Judith S. B. Guedalia and Frances R. Yoeli
SUMMARY SHEET BY MARILYN LUBER

Name: _____ Diagnosis: _____

Medications: _____

Test Results: _____

Date: _____

Phase 1: History Taking

Screening

Shows basic level of physical readiness:	☐ Completed _____ Time
Focuses eyes:	☐ Completed _____ Time
Responds to questions:	☐ Completed _____ Time
Looks around:	☐ Completed _____ Time
Shows interest in surroundings:	☐ Completed _____ Time
Breathing cadence slows to normal:	☐ Completed _____ Time
Connection to therapist:	☐ Completed _____ Time
Install sense of safety, trust, and realization they are alive:	☐ Completed _____ Time
Hysteria:	☐ Yes ☐ No _____ Time
Fugue-like state:	☐ Yes ☐ No _____ Time

Phase 2: Preparation

Permission to Touch: ☐ Yes ☐ No _____ Time

Neuropsychological Lesson ☐ Completed _____ Time

Say, "When we experience trauma, our brain takes in many sounds, feelings, images, smells, and even tastes, all at the same time. This avalanche of sensations coupled with the very real fear of dying, gets encoded or locked in our brain. The area of the brain that is generally activated in such situations is called the limbic system. This is the area that stores and processes emotion in our brain. This area experiences memories and is not generally seen as accessible by speech."

We use this further explanation to encourage the patient's recovery and cooperation.

Say, *"This is especially true soon after the event has occurred* (this seems to be a neuropsychological reality). *Initially trauma is a cortical experience in the limbic system, specifically the hippocampus. The hippocampus is an area of the brain that looks like a seahorse. It is responsible for episodic memory and spatial navigation. Unlike motor memory such as remembering how to ride a bicycle or swim or factual memory such as recalling dates of historical events, episodic memory involves day-today, short-term memories—what we did yesterday, or whom we met last week. It is the area that scientists now understand to be affected in traumatic experiences. What seems to occur is very visceral* (internal in the brain) *and is not neuropsychologically available for verbal encoding. The senses such as feeling, seeing, smelling, hearing, and taste are the modalities by which information is received, processed, and encoded by the brain. Research has shown* (and our clinical experience has found) *that before these images, smells, sounds, and so forth get stored, it is beneficial to talk and give words to these sensory inputs so as to allow them to be available for verbal access in the future."*

This may be very complicated and wordy for the ER patient. But the presence of the therapist's voice and the explanation, well understood or not, tends to foster a sense of calm and safety. In general, we begin this after the patient is somewhat stabilized. Also, it gives family members something to hang onto once we begin. They may be afraid of responses that we understand to be normal for Acute Stress Disorder (ASD) patients. Also, some aspects of the cognitive intervention may be understood and begin to help the patient formulate a frame of reference and then build on it in a logical scaffolding sort of way.

Phase 3: Assessment

Body language concerns: _____

_____

Agitation in vocabulary (NCs): _____

_____

Narrative: _____

_____
_____
_____
_____
_____
_____
_____
_____
_____
_____
_____
_____
_____

Target/Memory/Image of Actual Traumatic Event: _____

PC: _____

VoC: _____ /7

NC: _____

Emotions: _____
SUD: _____/10
Sensation: _____

Phase 4: Desensitization

Narrative: (2nd Time; Note Metaphors) ☐ Completed _____ Time

_____
_____
_____
_____
_____
_____
_____
_____
_____
_____
_____

BLS: _____ Hands _____ Knees _____ Shoulders
Homework:
  Count breaths: ☐ Completed _____ Time

Narrative: (3rd Time; Note Metaphors) ☐ Completed _____ Time

_____
_____
_____
_____
_____
_____
_____
_____
_____
_____
_____
_____

Emotions: _____

SUD: _____/10

Sensation: _____

Phase 5: Installation

Therapist builds sequence of events so there is a coherent narrative emphasizing survival
  Emotions: _____
  SUD: _____/10
  Sensation (only ask if NOT physically injured): _____

Able to verbalize sensory experience/
  coherent account with appropriate affect: ☐ Completed _____ Time
Able to get up off gurney, bed/chair: ☐ Completed _____ Time

Phase 6: Body Scan

Stopped uncontrollable crying: ☐ Completed _____ Time
More control of emotions: ☐ Completed _____ Time
Decrease of physical signs (uncontrollable shaking,
  perspiring, perseveration): ☐ Completed _____ Time
Lower cadence of speech: ☐ Completed _____ Time
Fuller breathing: ☐ Completed _____ Time
Narrative filled out: ☐ Completed _____ Time
Worrying about specifics (where is wallet?): ☐ Completed _____ Time
Hungry: ☐ Completed _____ Time
Unresolved/unprocessed information: _____

_____
_____
_____

Phase 7: Closure

Narrative: (Final Feedback) _____

_____
_____
_____
_____
_____
_____
_____
_____
_____
_____
_____
_____

Handout: ☐ Completed _____ Time

Social Services Consultation and Release:

Verified place to go: ☐ Completed _____ Time
Person picking patient up: ☐ Completed _____ Time
  Name of person: _____
Official release: ☐ Completed _____ Time

Phase 8: Reevaluation

Follow up:
  Hospital: ☐ Completed _____ Time of Appointment
_____

  Other: _____

EMDR Early Intervention Procedures for Individuals

What do we do when we are faced with a disaster? As a psychotherapy model, Eye Movement Desensitization and Reprocessing (EMDR) was conceptualized originally as a modality for individuals. In both of her texts on EMDR, Francine Shapiro (1995, 2001) began with having a standard protocol that focused on a traumatic memory. She was intrigued to discover that by finding an image that represented the entire memory or the worst part, other associations were activated relating to the traumatic memory network and adaptive ones, finally resulting in an integrated memory. Her new conceptualization (EMDR) was turning out to be a very helpful and exciting way to work with trauma.

In 1989, clients came in for treatment after the San Francisco Bay Area earthquake and Francine began to notice a difference in the way that her clients were presenting with their experiences of the earthquake. Now, when they would reprocess the most traumatic part of the memory, she found that the effects of the reprocessing were *not* generalizing to the other areas of the memory. It was as if each part had its own separate existence. It made her wonder about memory and how long one needed before it was assimilated and became an integrated experience. She thought that there was some level of consolidation because clients were able to tell what happened in a sequential manner but it turned out that there were no real links from one part of the memory to the next during this early time frame. From her observation, it was taking approximately 2 to 3 months for that to happen. She noted that one way for therapists to know that the consolidation of the recent traumatic memory was complete was when the Standard EMDR Protocol could be used successfully. If it was not possible, this new protocol, "Protocol for Recent Traumatic Events," was recommended. This protocol is scripted by this author from Francine's 2001 text and 2006 manual, *EMDR New Notes on Adaptive Information Processing With Case Formulation Principles, Forms, Scripts, and Worksheets*. In Francine's more extended protocol for recent trauma, she has seven steps; an eighth step was added to include Future Template—a step that she implies but did not officially mention in her books.

The Protocol for Recent Traumatic Events begins with a description of the event in narrative form, while the therapist notes the different elements of the experience. Each of these elements is targeted separately with the Standard EMDR Protocol up to the cognitive installation—but not including the body scan—until all of the targets have been reprocessed. The client is to start with the most disturbing part; if there is no particular disruptive aspect, then the suggestion is to start at the beginning of the event. When all of the elements are reprocessed, the clinician asks the client to close his eyes and experience the incident fully while visualizing the entire event as if he were sitting in a movie theater watching a film or at home viewing a TV show, without BLS. The goal is to see if there is any emotional, cognitive, or somatic charge during the viewing. If he is experiencing some distress, the client is to open his eyes and let his therapist know; the therapist then works with the client to reprocess this part of the memory, including accessing negative and positive cognitions. This is repeated until all is clear emotionally, cognitively, and somatically, and then the client is instructed to run though the event one more time with eyes open, including the positive cognition, and to signal with the stop sign when he is completed. When this part of the protocol is finished, a body scan is done. The next step is to target any triggers such as startle responses, nightmares, and other reminders of the incident that are still disturbing to the client. Then, a Future Template can be implemented. When all of these steps are finished, the event is considered processed. This is a powerful protocol and used a great deal.

As is always the case, when we begin to work with a basic protocol in the field, over time, new discoveries are made and suggestions to improve the procedure follow. Both Elan Shapiro and Brurit Laub live in Israel, and have developed their conceptualization of early EMDR intervention (EEI) and the Recent-Traumatic Episode Protocol (R-TEP) based on their work with clients during acute phases following war and terrorist-related issues, as well as motor vehicle accidents and other recent trauma. They hoped to capitalize on intervening before the consolidation of memory in a way to promote a client's recovery and resilience. Emphasizing that the aftermath of the traumatic event may be as or more important than the event itself, their idea of the "Traumatic Episode" includes targeting and reprocessing the disturbing fragments, experiences, and events from the original incident up until the present. In their EEI model, they fill out Francine's Protocol for Recent Traumatic Events by emphasizing the importance of the containment of the usually agitated client after recent trauma. They propose a way to quickly assess the readiness of the client to begin R-TEP processing during history taking using screening instruments.

During the Preparation Phase, they include the introduction of their own stabilization and resource exercises: Four Elements for Stress Management, including Safe Place (F. Shapiro, 2009, pp. 67–69) and Resource Connection (Laub, 2001, 2009, pp. 93–99).

In the R-TEP, unlike Francine's protocol, the narrative is accompanied by bilateral stimulation during Phase 3. Targets are referred to as Points of Disturbance (PoD) and found through an "Episode Google Search." There is an assessment of each PoD separately followed by processing, where they introduce the concept of "Telescopic Processing" with three optional strategies, referred to as EMD, EMDr, or EMDR strategies. Beginning with a recent trauma focus, usually with the EMDr strategy, or with an optional narrow EMD strategy advised for intrusive sensorimotor fragments, the full standard EMDR strategy is available when the former two circumscribed strategies are insufficient. Once the Trauma-Episode can be related to as a whole, Phases 5–8 follow.

In this way, Elan and Brurit can meet the clients where they are and target the fragment, the episode, and/or the theme, closely following their clients' needs. The main approach of the R-TEP is the EMDr strategy, where the associations relate just to the current traumatic episode. This is different than Francine's protocol, where each disturbing aspect of the memory is targeted with the EMDR protocol including the cognitions, with no concern stated to where the associations go. In R-TEP, anytime associations go beyond the episode they are asked to go Back To Target (BTT) and the SUDs are checked. In the EMD strategy, the associations are limited only to the PoD. The EMDR strategy with no censure on associations is only included when adaptive resolution of the episode is not reached. This will require clients' consent, as this was not the original agreement when they came in for recent trauma treatment.

In R-TEP, clients do a Google Search/scan instead of doing a visualization of the entire sequence of the event with eyes closed and then open until the event can be visualized without charge. As in Francine's work, negative cognitions can relate to the situation and not the self. If future targets are expressed, they are reprocessed in the same way as other targets. When the SUD level of the PoD is ecological, an installation is performed in the usual way. They note the importance of having a strong closure at the finish of each session. An installation—as with Francine's work—is installed also for the entire episode. The R-TEP is completed for the most part when all of the PoDs have been processed, the Episode PC has been installed, and the session is closed down using already developed resources. On follow up, if the Episode-SUD is not 0, then another Google Search ensues until the target/s have no change.

In Chapter 4, "The EMDR Protocol for Recent Critical Incidents (EMDR-PRECI)," developed by Ignacio Jarero (Nacho) and Lucina (Lucy) Artigas—who were introduced in earlier sections—also modified Francine's Protocol for Recent Traumatic Events after their years of involvement in Latin America and the Caribbean. Their modifications grew out of the need to treat clients after critical incidents occured, but where other related disturbing events continue over a long period of time and where there is no post-trauma period of safety for memory consolidation. For example, when they were working with the forensic personnel who had the task of body recovery for the State Attorney General of the Mexican state of Durango subsequent to finding seven graves holding the murdered corpses, victims of drug warfare (Jarero, Artigas, & Luber, 2011; Jarero & Uribe, 2011, 2012). The reason that the length of time became important was because they saw the phenomena that Francine saw after the 1989 earthquake, except they observed that even 6 months after the event, their clients' memories seemed like the unconsolidated recent traumatic event. They realized that acute trauma situations are not only related to the time frame in days or months, but also to what they call a "post-trauma safety period." They maintain that it is this lack of a post-trauma period of safety that is what is preventing the consolidation of the memory of the original trauma. This is because there are continuing stressful events with similar enough information such as emotions, physical sensations, etc., that do not give the state-dependent traumatic memory enough time to ever consolidate into an integrated whole. In this way, the memory network is permanently activated and expands with each new stressful experience that occurs. As a result, concentrating on one part of the memory does not generalize to the whole memory during reprocessing (Jarero et al., 2011). This was a very important finding.

During the History-Taking Phase, the EMDR-PRECI conceptualizes the incident as an extended event with a continuum of ongoing stressful events; therefore, clients are asked to tell the narrative from right before the incident until the present. Francine conceptualizes the traumatic event as comprised of a number of separate moments within an event while the R-TEP sees the traumatic episode as the traumatic incident and its aftermath like a trauma continuum from just before the original incident until the present, comprised of a number of targets of disturbing fragments, experiences, and events, but discourages going into much detail at this stage so as to avoid premature activation. There is no BLS used during this phase for any of the protocols. However, in the R-TEP, the detailed account of the trauma episode is elicited later, together with BLS, for dual attention grounding, containment, and initial processing as part of the treatment.

In the EMDR-PRECI, they introduce the self-administered Butterfly Hug during the Preparation Phase as a way to empower clients, whereas the other protocols use therapist-generated BLS. They include their own self-soothing techniques: Abdominal Breathing, the Concentration Exercise, and/or Pleasant Memory Technique.

During their Assessment Phase, they have clients mentally run a movie of the episode before it occurred until the present and then ask for the worst part. They are not as concerned with the negative cognition; however, they will attempt to elicit one and offer, "I'm in danger," if none is forthcoming. Unlike the other two protocols, they do not elicit a PC or VoC, since their thought is that the stressful situation may make it more difficult for them to find PCs during the Assessment Phase.

During the Desensitization Phase, as with the other protocols, the target is processed; however, the Installation Phase is not done for fragments as it is done in the other protocols.

When this first target is completed, they ask clients to visualize the complete sequence of events with eyes closed to find any remaining fragments with disturbance; then, they process them with image, NC, emotion, and SUD, but not the PC or VoC. In Francine's protocol, any remaining disturbing events are processed in chronological order, then the client is asked to visualize the event with eyes closed to find any remaining disturbance; the full Assessment Phase is used for each moment found. While in R-TEP, after the PoD is processed a Google search is used with continuous BLS to find another Point of Disturbance, but not necessarily in chronological order.

It is only when there are no further disturbances identified that a PC is developed for the entire event, without frequent checking of the VoC. Although the other two protocols ask for a representative PC for the extended event and link it with the entire event while doing BLS also, they engage in frequent checking of the VoC. At this point, the EMDR-PRECI inserts a Supplement Step and asks, with eyes closed, to think of the PC and review the whole sequence. At the end, the following question is asked: "Does the PC feel less true on any part of the sequence?" If so, the part is targeted.

Phases 6 and 7, and the 3-pronged approach, are all done according to the Standard EMDR Protocol and they use the already-learned self-soothing techniques to make sure that the Closure Phase is adequately done.

These chapters each have companion summary sheets for data entry and a brief exposition of the primary elements of the material.

Each of these protocols developed according to the observations of skilled professionals, who were actively engaged in the treatment of clients who experienced recent trauma. Their modifications reflect what they believed was needed to enhance their work and support the healing process within their clients. These protocols are beginning to be researched; time will tell concerning the robustness of these works. In the meantime, the observations that these authors and members of the EMDR community are finding is that the victims of man-made and natural disasters are better able to handle what other difficult obstacles befall them after they have processed their disaster targets. In a world where there is a surfeit of disasters and too little mental health response, these protocols aimed at reprocessing recent trauma are a step closer to creating a tidal wave of opportunity for healing those victims suffering from man-made and natural disasters.

# The Recent Traumatic Episode Protocol (R-TEP): An Integrative Protocol for Early EMDR Intervention (EEI)

Elan Shapiro and Brurit Laub

Early EMDR Intervention (EEI)

The question of how early to intervene with EMDR in the face of natural and man-made disasters has been an important part of the dialogue of those working in this field. As a result of the human beings suffering in the wake of these catastrophes, a number of ideas have ensued and new ways to work with the pain and anguish have been explored. Whereas the majority of people who experience a significant trauma will recover spontaneously, there is often prolonged suffering and about one-third may be left with enduring distressing clinical or subclinical symptoms of posttraumatic stress disorder (PTSD) and other psychiatric disorders (National Institute for Clinical Excellence [NICE], 2005).

Early EMDR intervention (EEI), before consolidation of the memory has taken place, may reduce associative connections to past traumas, preventing the accumulation of traumatic memories. It may also enhance adaptive associations, promoting adaptive integration reflected in self-affirmation, coping, resilience, and other measures of "post-traumatic growth." Therefore, early EMDR intervention should be considered following a significant trauma. How and when to intervene with EEI most effectively and whether it can thereby reduce the incidence of PTSD and other disorders that can follow trauma are among the challenges that need to be studied empirically.

Informed by the work of Francine Shapiro, Roger Solomon, and all of the friends and colleagues in the field who have contributed to the evolution of their thinking and practice and following clinical and empirical experience with early EMDR intervention in the wake of the 2006 Lebanon war, the authors have observed that the existing EEI protocols appear to focus on certain aspects or parts of the traumatic episode along an approximate time line continuum following a trauma, in accordance with the *Diagnostic and Statistical Manual of Mental Disorders (DSM-5)* (American Psychiatric Association [APA], 2013). They concluded that the unfinished processing of recent traumatic events may require a broader approach than existing early EMDR intervention (EEI) protocols provided.

Looking at the existing protocols, Shapiro and Laub (2008) suggest that the earliest interventions (e.g., emergency room protocols) that use elements of EMDR, such as Bilateral Stimulation (BLS), are primarily used for calming and stabilization for Acute Stress Response (ASR). The EMD Protocol is most effectively used for processing intrusive sensorimotor fragments. The protocol for Recent Traumatic Events (RTE) is used for processing an unconsolidated discrete event and the Standard EMDR Protocol is used to process memories that are already consolidated in a theme cluster. However, they suggest that the original traumatic incident and its aftermath may be conceived more like an ongoing *trauma continuum* while the experiences have not yet been consolidated. They propose a new protocol called the Recent-Traumatic Episode Protocol (R-TEP), which incorporates and extends the existing EEI protocols by providing a new comprehensive, integrative protocol. The R-TEP thus bridges the gaps left by previous protocols and facilitates a transition from the EMD and RE protocols to the Standard EMDR Protocol.

The R-TEP takes the wisdom of the Standard EMDR Protocol (Shapiro, 1995, 2001), and applies it in an adapted form for recent events to provide a comprehensive approach to Early EMDR Intervention. It is a protocol that adapts the EMD and the Recent Event Protocols within a newly conceived extended time perspective, termed here the "Traumatic Episode." The Traumatic Episode (or T-Episode) comprises a number of targets of disturbing fragments and experiences (images, sensations, feelings, and thoughts) in the trauma continuum, from the original incident until the present, which need to be processed.

New theoretical conceptualizations of the process of memory consolidation, relating to Francine Shapiro's Adaptive Information Processing (AIP) model (Shapiro, 1995, 2001), guided the development of the R-TEP. It is suggested that the stages of this process proceed hierarchically according to part/whole relations aiming toward adaptive integration (see Figure 1). This integrative sequence is of a broadening focus from the intrusive image/sensation fragment to the event, to the episode that includes many events, to the theme, and to the identity that is comprised of clusters of themes. When a part (such as an intrusive fragment) is stuck (blocked/dissociated or locked/re-experienced), the AIP system is disrupted and cannot move toward the next whole, and thus fails to reach integration. Information is transmitted at increasing levels of complexity, from the sensorimotor (sensory and somatic) to the experiential (sensorimotor and emotional) and to the meaning (sensorimotor, emotional, and cognitive) levels, perhaps matching the evolution of the brain. It is assumed that the AIP system moves toward integration dialectically via associative connections between the various opposites of the traumatic memory networks and the adaptive ones (horizontal dialectical movement) going through part/whole integrative sequences (vertical dialectical movement) (Laub & Weiner, 2011).

The R-TEP employs an adapted eight-phase structure, with some modifications for application to early EMDR intervention. These modifications are based on the fragmented nature of the memory, on the need for containment and safety, and the wider T-Episode time frame. The T-Episode is conceived as a continuum from the original incident to the present and anticipated future concerns.

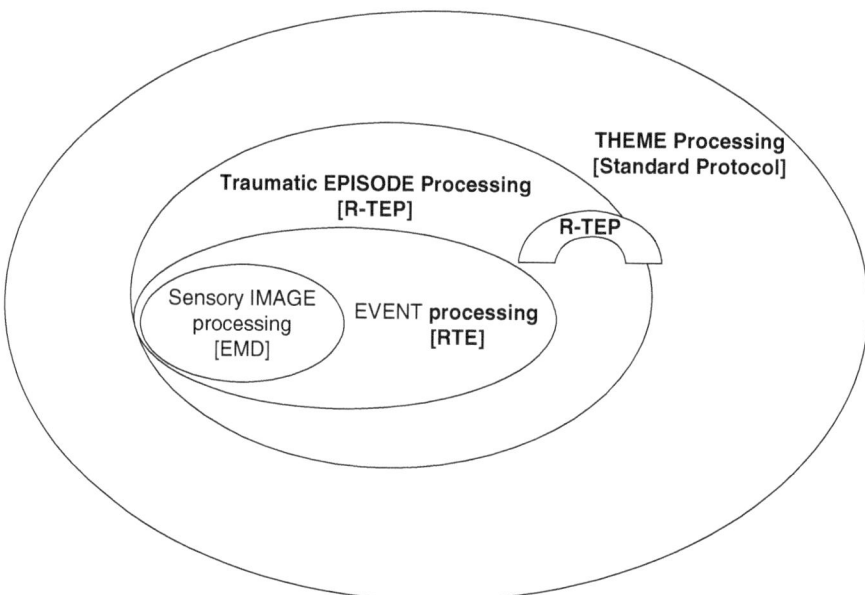

Figure 1   R-TEP (Recent-Traumatic Episode Protocol). Part/whole integrative sequence of the memory consolidation process after recent trauma—a bridge from episode to theme processing in early (EMDR) interventions (EEI) (Shapiro & Laub, 2008).

Main Issues in Early EMDR Intervention (EEI)

Clinical experience indicates that EMDR can be beneficial for alleviating excessive distress and complications in the weeks and months following critical events. However, there seems to be uncertainty and inconsistency among many clinicians about which protocols to use for Early EMDR Intervention and how and when to use them. Consequently, there is a need for a comprehensive model and set of guidelines in the EMDR practitioner's toolbox to assist in approaching the prospect of EEI with more confidence and to generate research.

Issues to consider when working with EEI:

1. *Memory:* In recent trauma the nature of the memory is fragmented and not consolidated; it requires a different protocol.
2. *When to Intervene:* When there is distress, particularly when it is clinically significant, when to intervene is straightforward. However, when symptoms are subclinical, the question to ask is, "Is prevention to be considered?" Reference is made to the literature on delayed-onset and sensitization (Andrews, Brewin, Philpott, & Stewart, 2007; McFarlane, 2010).
3. *Therapeutic Situation:* The nature of the situation for client and therapist is that there is an atmosphere of emergency or urgency that often results in high arousal or distress and sometimes avoidance; this requires a special attention to containment and safety.
4. *Therapy Contract:* The nature of the therapy contract may be unclear, and as a result professional and ethical standards may be compromised; this requires good practice guidelines. The R-TEP attempts to address these issues within the protocol as a comprehensive approach to EEI.

The Recent-Traumatic Episode Protocol Features

Main Features of R-TEP

1. A comprehensive approach to EEI: The eight phases.
2. An integrative approach to EEI: Incorporates adaptations of the EMD and RE protocols.
3. The Traumatic-Episode (T-Episode): This is a newly conceived trauma continuum time frame.
4. The Google-Search (G-Search): This is a procedure for scanning and identifying targets of disturbance or Point of Disturbance (PoD) within the T-Episode.
5. "Telescopic Processing": Suggests three optional strategies for the processing in Phase 4 (Desensitization) for a contained intervention with varying boundaries for the chains of associations. Advocating a current trauma focus, the EMD strategy provides a narrow focus on the disturbing fragment; the EMDr strategy enables a broader focus on the current trauma episode; or (only if necessary and with client consent), the EMDR strategy that relates to the whole of life experiences.
6. Special attention to containment and safety.
7. Maintaining standards of good practice.
8. Theoretical underpinning.

Adapted Eight Phases of the R-TEP

This novel application of the eight-phase framework for EEI provides a structure that fosters safety and maintains professional standards of good practice even in recent event situations where they risk being compromised. The eight phases follow the Standard EMDR Protocol, but they are divided into three groupings to emphasize the specific features of the R-TEP:

A. Episode history taking and preparation (often neglected in EEI)
  1. Phase 1 : History-Taking/Intake
     To assess readiness for EEI.

2. Phase 2: Preparation
      To attend to safety, containment and gaining some self-stabilization and control
 B. Point of Disturbance (PoD) Level of Processing
    To identify, assess, and process disturbing targets.
    1. Traumatic-Episode narrative with continuous Bilateral Stimulation (BLS)
       To tell the story of the traumatic episode out loud with BLS
    2. "Episode Google Search"
       To identify Points of Disturbance relating to the T-Episode from the original incident until today, including all the related events and disturbances.
    3. Assessment of each PoD in turn that becomes the target fragment, using as much of the Standard EMDR Protocol assessment as appropriate (use clinical judgment)
    4. "Telescopic Processing"
       The term "Telescopic Processing" is used to reflect the three optional strategies for Phase 4 Desensitization: (EMD < > EMDr .... EMDR) following the memory consolidation process after recent trauma.
 C. Episode Level—the Trauma-Episode is related to as a whole
    1. Check Episode Subjective Unit of Disturbance (SUD)
    2. Episode Level Phase 5: Installation of Episode Positive Cognition (PC)
    3. Episode Level Phase 6: Episode Body Scan
    4. Phase 7: Closure of the Episode
    5. Phase 8: Follow Up

The Google Search (G-Search)

The Google Search (G-Search) is a metaphor for a scanning procedure to identify targets of disturbance within the T-Episode. It identifies Points of Disturbance targets non-sequentially, in a natural associative way. Each target is identified from the entire episode and processed (usually about three or four targets in two to four sessions, optionally on consecutive days), to reach adaptive resolution. When there are no more targets identified at this Points of Disturbance level, go to the Episode level of the entire Trauma-Episode, which includes the Episode PC and Installation, Body Scan, and Closure; this is usually quite a short procedure.

The (recent) past traumatic incident influences our sense of safety and control in the present as well as our future expectations. Therefore, concerns about the future arising during the G-Search may also be important targets for processing.

Special Attention to Containment and Safety

In addition to the containment and safety provided by the adapted eight phase framework and the stabilization and resources exercise in the Preparation Phase, there are some other measures.

Episode Narrative

During Phases 1 and 2, the client is deliberately not asked to recount the details of the trauma yet, except in general terms, so as to avoid prematurely triggering abreaction and possible re-traumatization before containment and safety measures are in place and treatment processing can begin. The Trauma-Episode Narrative is carried out adding BLS during the telling of the story with an optional distancing technique. This appears to increase the sense of safety because of the presumed grounding and de-arousal effects of the BLS.

Telescopic Processing: A Three Strategies Approach
(EMD <—> EMDr With Optional EMDR)

The possibility of using three strategies with different boundaries for chains of associations can provide contained processing. The narrow focused EMD processing allows a brief and contained processing of intrusive fragments that may block the AIP system. The boundaries

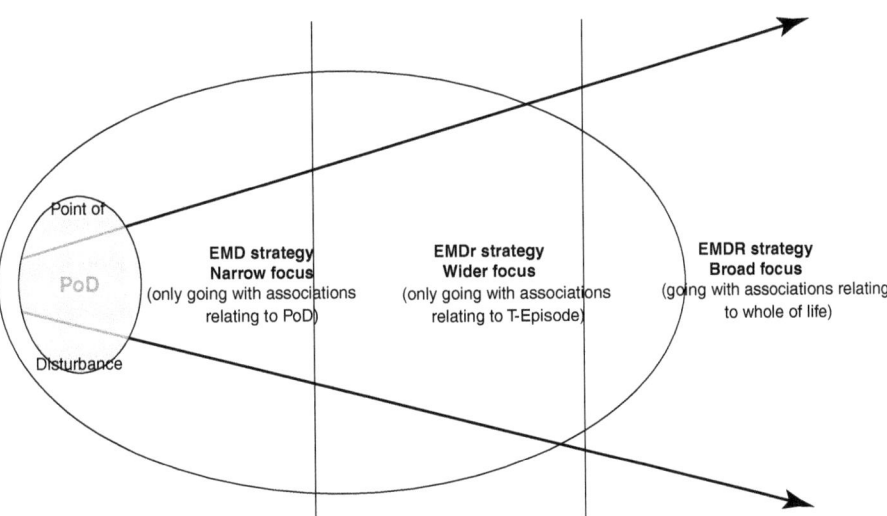

Figure 2 R-TEP "Telescopic Processing." Three optional strategies of a broadening focus: EMD, EMDr, or EMDR. (From Shapiro & Laub, 2011.)

in EMDr processing with associations predominantly relating to the current trauma episode discourages opening past channels that may overload, while acknowledging their possible relevance; thus, differentiation between past and present is encouraged, thereby allowing a more contained processing.

Guidelines for Maintaining Standards of Good Practice With R-TEP

In the unusual circumstances of EEI, there are a number of risks that should be noted to ensure optimal EMDR therapy practice. There are various opinions about early psychological intervention and there is no intervention yet which evidence-based practice has endorsed for routine intervention (Roberts, Kitchiner, Kenardy, & Bisson, 2009, for the Cochrane review). There are legitimate concerns about premature intervention, fear of causing harm, short cuts, and coping with affect containment.

Prior History. The way in which the clinician intervenes in EEI needs to be considered. In general, the clinician will encounter normal people who have been exposed to abnormal situations. However some of them will have previous histories of pathology, dysfunction, or trauma. Specifically, care should be taken to avoid common pitfalls such as: excessive shortcuts in Phases 1 (insufficient history, intake, ego strength assessment) and 2 (insufficient rapport and preparation), as well as opening other clinical issues when this is not part of the therapy contract (in EMDR you know where you start but not where you may go).

Traumatic Episode. When possible, give priority to focusing on the traumatic episode and its concomitants, and only go into other clinical issues that arise if this is not sufficient to promote adaptive processing. While we need to be flexible in these circumstances, we also need to bear in mind our professional boundaries and standards when working with recent trauma.

Timing of Intervention. The question of when to intervene is still an open question and there are various opinions of when to intervene.

Guidelines for When to Intervene

In General. When Psychological First Aid is not sufficient, when there is excessive suffering and persistent disturbing symptoms, especially intrusive images and sleep disturbance, when high risk is evaluated, and/or when preventive action is possible.

Hours After Trauma. In addition to Psychological First Aid, consider first using the Emergency Response Procedure (ERP) for stabilizing and calming, an alternative to medication (see Chapter 1).

Days After Trauma. Use R-TEP with a likely focus on brief EMD for intrusions and sleep disturbance.

Weeks and Months After Trauma. Use R-TEP with focus on EMDr for treatment of traumatic stress and/or prevention of accumulation of trauma memories and sensitization (see McFarlane, 2010).

The R-TEP proposes a current trauma episode focused therapy contract. However, the Standard EMDR Protocol is always available for use when the EMDr and EMD strategies are not sufficient for adaptively processing the current trauma episode and previous trauma or blocking beliefs need to be considered. This requires client consent.

The R-TEP, therefore, embodies a set of guidelines, with built-in safeguards for checking one's work and maintaining standards of good practice in line with the Standard EMDR Protocol.

The Recent-Traumatic Episode Protocol (R-TEP) Notes

2013 Update: Note the changes in the guidelines for Telescopic Processing Phase 4 Desensitization strategies.*

Phase 1 : Client History/Intake

Obtain as much client history and information as possible in the circumstances to screen for previous pathology. Administer the Impact of Events Scale (IES-R) when possible, to obtain a baseline measure prior to intervention as part of the assessment and again post intervention to assess effectiveness. Then, estimate Severity, Motivation, and Strengths (SMS] ratings on a 5-point scale (1 = low to 5 = high) in order to decide whether it is appropriate to proceed with EMDR processing with the client at this time. Minimum strengths and motivation ratings of 3 are advocated to proceed when the severity is high.

A summary of SMS ratings based on all information obtained and clinical impression is listed.

S = Severity	(low)	1	2	3	4	5 (high)
M = Motivation	(low)	1	2	3	4	5 (high)
S = Strengths	(low)	1	2	3	4	5 (high)

Phase 2: Preparation

In early EMDR intervention, clients are likely to be easily flooded with states of high arousal and distress. Therefore, Phase 2 Preparation is particularly important for establishing sufficient safety, containment, and some sense of control to enable EMDR processing.

In all cases, start with stabilization and resource exercises for calming and enhancing control such as: The Four Elements for Stress Management, Safe Place (E. Shapiro, 2009a, pp. 67–69), and Resource Connection (Laub, 2001, 2009, pp. 93–99). Write down the exercises or scripts used for each of these.

During Phases 1 and 2, the client is deliberately not asked to recount the details of the trauma yet, except in general terms, so as to avoid triggering abreaction and possible re-traumatization before containment and safety measures are in place and treatment processing can begin.

Point of Disturbance (PoD) Level of Processing (Phases 3, 4 ,5, and 7)

These phases include assessment and processing of the targets identified in the traumatic episode, from the original incident until today, including disturbing thoughts about the future.

The goal of episode processing is to integrate the intrusive fragments and other disturbing experiences of the Trauma Episode into an adaptive episode that is finally integrated into the autobiographical story of the individual.

1. *Episode Narrative With Bilateral Stimulation (BLS)*
   In the Episode Narrative, the client tells the story of the traumatic episode out loud with BLS, which helps to ground and contain affect. It is the first time that the client tells the traumatic story in a sequential and detailed way in the presence of an empathic witnessing therapist. It seems that this procedure entails an initial processing, though more verbal and conscious than Telescopic Processing, which brings about an initial sense of integration. Using a distancing metaphor, such as a TV screen, gives additional containment if needed.
2. *Episode "Google Search" (or G-Search) With BLS*
   Note: For clients who may not understand the Google Search metaphor, just say, "Scan."
3. For the assessment of each PoD in turn, use as much of the Standard EMDR Protocol assessment as appropriate (when there is high arousal and/or the PoD is an activating intrusion, flexibility is advised and a partial assessment may be conducted).
4. *Telescopic Processing*
   Provides boundaries for focused contained processing: the EMD strategy for a narrow PoD focus and the EMDr strategy for a broader current trauma episode focus. The EMDR strategy of the Standard EMDR Protocol is used if the other two strategies were not sufficient to reach adaptive resolution.
   - *****EMDr strategy:** This is the main strategy of Telescopic Processing. In this strategy the associative span relates *to the current traumatic episode*. If an association comes up—which is not related to the traumatic episode—it is acknowledged but the client is asked to re-focus by going Back To Target (BTT) to the PoD and checking the SUD.
   - *****EMD strategy:** Narrow focused processing limiting the range of associations to those related only to the PoD. This is a brief strategy, particularly effective with intrusive image/sensation fragments. If the association is not directly related to the PoD, the client is asked gently to re-focus by going BTT and checking the SUD frequently.
     The EMD strategy is suggested in the following situations:
     a. When the target/PoD is an intrusive element fragment (frequently recurring disturbing image, sensation, thought, feeling). However, if the SUD is not reducing significantly after about six sets, then expand naturally into the EMDr strategy.
     b. When there is still an intrusive/painful fragment that blocks the AIP system, or when the SUD level is not reducing with the EMDr strategy, consider narrowing to an EMD strategy, in addition to Interweaves Procedure, which can be attempted to get the processing moving
   - **EMDR strategy:** This is the widest focus. It is only used, if necessary, to include the whole span of life with no limitation of associations, according to the Standard EMDR Protocol. It requires the client's consent, as the initial contract is the current trauma focus. This step is optional and rare.

The Recent Traumatic Episode Protocol Script

Explanation of R-TEP

This is the introduction to the R-TEP given to the client:

Say, *"This EMDR protocol is especially suited for early intervention. Its aim is to help your natural processing system process the disturbing fragments of the traumatic episode so that you can restore your balance. Let whatever comes to mind come up. Sometimes, I will ask you to go back to a certain part of the memory, and sometimes not. At other times, we might note something that we could come back to later, if we choose, then we will refocus on the current traumatic episode.*

It is like zooming in, or zooming out, which can help you focus on, observe, and process your memories and experiences, so that the past and present are not confused, and you can begin feeling calmer, safer, and more in control."

Episode Narrative Script

In the Episode narrative, the client tells the story of the traumatic incident out loud with EMDR.

Say, *"Do you feel* (relatively) *comfortable and safe here now in this room?"*

_____
_____

If the answer is no, then more preparation and stabilization is needed first.

Say, *"I am going to ask you to view the whole T-Episode, beginning a few minutes before it started until today. Feel your feet on the ground, the safety of this room, and tell the story out loud. "*

If this is too close for the client, suggest the following:

Say, *"I am going to ask you to view the whole T-Episode, beginning a few minutes before it started until today. Feel your feet on the ground, the safety of this room and tell the story out loud and watch the whole episode as on TV. Imagine that you are watching the episode on a screen with a remote control that can make the screen smaller, farther away, lower the volume, or even pause it. "*

Use continuous BLS during the Episode narrative.

_____
_____
_____
_____
_____
_____
_____

Episode Google Search Script

In the Google Search Script, the client searches for anything disturbing, and in no particular order.

Say, *"Now, without talking out loud this time, return to scan the whole episode-like a Google Search in the computer—for anything that is disturbing, and in no particular order. Just notice what comes up as you search the whole episode from the original event until today and stop at what is disturbing you."*

Use continuous BLS during the G-Search.

_____
_____

Assess (Phase 3) the target of the identified PoD (intrusive fragment or more complex experience). Target and process each PoD (intrusive fragments and other experiences of the events within the episode). For Phase 3, use as much of the Standard EMDR Protocol assessment as appropriate such as NC, PC, VoC, Emotion, SUD, and Body Sensation. During the

Telescopic Processing (Phase 4: Desensitization), use mostly the EMDr Strategy. If the PoD is an intrusive fragment use the EMD strategy. During EMDr, if processing is stuck because of an intrusive fragment, consider using the EMD Strategy.

Phase 3: Assessment

Target

Say, *"Describe the disturbance"*

_____
_____

If the PoD is not an image, access a picture associated with it.

Say, *"When you focus on the _____ (state the PoD), what picture comes in mind?"*

_____
_____

Negative Cognition (NC)

Say, *"What negative words go with that _____ (state the PoD) about yourself now?"*

_____
_____

A negative cognition related to the situation and not to the self is accepted. If there is high arousal or difficulty in rapidly finding an NC, suggest a suitable NC. Clients usually speak about physical survival categories of safety or control in these types of situations, such as, *"I'm in danger," "I am helpless,"* and *"It shouldn't happen."*

Positive Cognition (PC)

Say, *"When you bring up that _____ (state PoD), how would you like to think about it, or about yourself?"*

_____
_____

If it is difficult to find a PC, while the level of disturbance is high, offer a tentative PC that is appropriate to the NC.

Say, *"Would you like to believe that 'It happened and it's over,' 'T survived,' 'I am safe now from THAT event,' and 'T can cope'? Is that what you would like to believe or is there something else you prefer?"*

_____
_____

Validity of Cognition (VoC)

You can skip the VoC, if it is not appropriate to ask at this stage.

Say, *"On a scale of 1 to 7, where 1 is completely false and 7 is completely true, how true do these words feel to you now?"*

1   2   3   4   5   6   7
[completely false]   (completely true)

Emotions

Say, *"When you bring up that _____ (state PoD) and those words (state the negative cognition), what emotion do you feel now?"*

_____

_____

Subjective Units of Disturbance (SUD)

Say, *"On a scale of 0 to 10, where 0 is bringing up the PoD and staying relatively calm and 10 is the highest disturbance you can imagine, how disturbing does the image feel to you now?"*

0   1   2   3   4   5   6   7   8   9   10
(no disturbance)   (highest disturbance)

Location of Body Sensation

Say, *"Where do you feel it in your body?"*

Phase 4: Telescopic Processing (Desensitization)

When working with R-TEP in the Telescopic Processing/Desensitization Phase, follow these guidelines:

1. Begin (usually) with the main EMDr strategy by focusing on chains of associations relating directly to the current Traumatic Episode.
2. When an intrusive image/sensation/emotion or thought is identified consider using the narrow-focused EMD strategy: short chains of associations relating only to the disturbing fragment (PoD).
3. Only if the first two strategies are not sufficient then consider employing the Standard EMDR Protocol with free associations related to the whole of life experiences, as in unlimited chains of associations. This is a clinical choice point that requires client consent.

EMDr Strategy for R-TEP Script

EMDr is the main strategy of the Telescopic Processing.

1. If the association is about the T-Episode:
   Say, *"Go with that."*

Continue with BLS and chains of associations as long as the association is related to the episode.

2. If the association is not about the T-Episode:

Say, *"We can note that, but as we have agreed to focus on the episode, I will ask you now to go back to the original disturbance_____(state the PoD). What do you get now?"*

_____

_____

Say, *"On a scale of 0 to 10, where 0 is bringing up the PoD and staying relatively calm and 10 is the highest disturbance you can imagine, how disturbing does it feel now?"*

0   1   2   3   4   5   6   7   8   9   10
(no disturbance)   (highest disturbance)

Continue the processing in this way until the SUD level drops to an ecological level or the target (PoD) can be viewed calmly. Then, proceed to the Installation Phase (see the Standard EMDR Protocol Script below).

Choice Point: If the SUD level still is not reducing or processing gets stuck, do another Google Search for another PoD. If processing is stuck, then, using your clinical judgment and with the client's consent, consider using the Standard EMDR Protocol.

Phase 5: Installation of the PoD

During assessment, a tentative PC was offered. An opportunity is given to find a more suitable PC now that the SUD has reduced.

Say, *"How does_____(repeat the PC) sound?"*

_____

Say, *"Do the words_____(state the PC) still fit, or is there another positive statement that you feel would be more suitable?"*

_____

If the client accepts the original positive cognition, the clinician should ask for a VoC rating to see if it has improved.

Validity of Cognition (VoC)

Say, *"As you think of the_____(state the original disturbance/PoD) and those words_____ (repeat the selected PC), how true do they feel, from 1 (completely false) to 7 (completely true)?"*

1   2   3   4   5   6   7
[completely false]   (completely true)

Say, *"Go with that."*

Do BLS. Then say the following:

Say, *"Think of the_____ (state the PoD), and hold it together with the words_____(repeat the PC)."*

Continue installation, with brief BLS, as long as the VoC strengthens.

Note: There is no Phase 6: Body Scan at this PoD Level of Processing as this is just one target of several.

Continue with the Episode G-Search, as before, to check if there are any other PoDs left and process similarly with Telescopic Processing.

Say, *"Now, again, without talking out loud, return to scan the whole episode, like a Google Search on the computer, for anything else that is disturbing you, in no particular order. Just notice what comes up as you search the whole episode from the original event until today and stop at what is still disturbing you and we will use it as a target for processing."*

Use continuous BLS during the G-Search.

___

Process any additional identified targets (PoDs) using Telescopic Processing. Repeat until there are no more targets.

When an intrusive image/sensation/emotion or thought is identified, consider using the narrow-focused EMD strategy.

EMD Strategy for R-TEP Script (Adapted From the EMD Protocol, Shapiro, 1995)

The EMD strategy limits associations. If associations relate directly to the PoD, the processing is continued. If associations depart from the PoD, then there is a return to Target (the PoD), and the SUD level is checked. A distancing metaphor can be suggested to help with high arousal if needed. It is usually a brief procedure, so if the SUD is not reducing after about six sets, "Zoom Out" smoothly to a wider EMDr strategy.

Say, *"I'd like you to bring up that_____(state the PoD), those negative words_____(state the negative cognition), and notice where you are feeling it in your body. Go with that."*

Ask the client to indicate when he wants to rest and stop the set.

Do a set of BLS. Sets could be short if client is in a high arousal.

After the set, say the following:

Say, *"Take a deep breath. What do you get now?"*

___

If the association is within the boundaries of the PoD continue.

Say, *"Go on."*

If the association departs from the PoD, go back to target (PoD)

Say, *"I would like to ask you to focus again on the_____(state the PoD) so you may digest it. Do you notice any change?"*

___

Say, *"On a scale of 0 to 10, where 0 is bringing up the PoD and staying relatively calm and 10 is the highest disturbance you can imagine, how disturbing does it feel now?"*

0   1   2   3   4   5   6   7   8   9   10
(no disturbance)   (highest disturbance)

Do another set of BLS.

Say, *"What do you get now?"*

___

If the association is within the boundaries of the PoD continue.

Say, *"Go with that."*

If the association departs from the PoD, go back to target (PoD).

Say, *"Let's go back again to the____(state the PoD). On a scale of 0 to 10, where 0 is accessing the PoD and staying relatively calm and 10 is the highest disturbance you can imagine, how disturbing does it feel now?"*

0   1   2   3   4   5   6   7   8   9   10
(no disturbance)   (highest disturbance)

Continue for about 6 to 10 sets until the SUD level reduces to ecological validity or when the original target can be viewed relatively calmly. Then proceed to installation of the PoD. If there is no change after about six sets, zoom out to EMDr strategy.

Note: If the SUD level is not reducing after about six sets, proceed without interrupting the flow (and without a new assessment), with a transition to the EMDr strategy (see above), which widens the focus of associations to the current traumatic episode.

Future Targets

Concerns about the future such as, *"What if it happens again?,"* a disrupted sense of personal safety, and challenges to the client's basic assumptions may arise during the G-Search. These future targets are processed in the same way as other targets. This may be helpful for strengthening resilience.

Since the T-Episode is comprised of several targets, the G-Search can be used over several sessions.

Ensure a strong closure at the end of each session using the Four Elements Exercise and/or a Resource Connection.

Episode Level

Checking the Episode-SUD (E-SUD)

When no more targets emerge with G-Search, check the SUD level for the entire T-Episode.

Say, *"When you think of the entire episode now, how disturbing is it to you on a scale of 0 to 10, where 0 is staying relatively calm and 10 is the highest disturbance you can imagine?"*

0   1   2   3   4   5   6   7   8   9   10
(no disturbance)   (highest disturbance)

When the SUD is ecological, proceed to installation of the Episode PC.

Phase 5: Installation of Episode Positive Cognition (E-PC)

Obtain a PC for the *entire* episode.

Say, *"When you think about the entire episode, how would you like to think about it now? What have you learned from it?"*

_____

_____

_____

Obtain a PC for the *entire* episode. Check the VoC.

Say, *"As you think of the entire episode again, how do the words*____(state the E-PC) *feel, from 1* (completely false) *to 7* (completely true)?"

1 2 3 4 5 6 7
[completely false]   (completely true)

Say, *"Hold them together, the entire episode and these words*____(repeat the E-PC)*".*

Install with sets of BLS and check the VoC.

Say, *"As you think of the entire episode again, how do the words*____(state the E-PC) *feel, from 1* (completely false) *to 7* (completely true)?"

1 2 3 4 5 6 7
[completely false]   (completely true)

Continue installation until it no longer changes and the VoC is 6 or 7. If the VoC is less than 7, say the following:

Say, *"What prevents this from being a 6 or 7?"*

_____

Do BLS.

Say, *"Go with that."*

Phase 6: Episode-Body Scan (This Is the Only Time the Body Scan Is Requested)

Say, *"When you think of the entire episode and your positive cognition*_____ (state E-PC), *notice any body sensations. Go with that."*

_____

Use sets of BLS as in the Standard EMDR Protocol.

Phase 7: Closure of the Episode

At this stage, after all the PoDs have been processed and the Episode PC has been installed, a supportive soft closure is suggested (e.g., a closing resource).

Phase 8: Follow Up

Check the Episode SUD Level.

Say, *"On a scale of 0 to 10, where 0 is bringing up the entire episode and staying calm with no disturbance or neutral and 10 is the highest disturbance you can imagine, how disturbing does the entire episode feel now?"*

0 1 2 3 4 5 6 7 8 9 10
(no disturbance)   (highest disturbance)

If the SUD does not equal 0 or does not seem ecological, use G-Search to identify any residual targets that may require additional processing.

Say, *"Now, again, without talking out loud, return to scan the whole episode, like a Google Search on the computer, for anything else that is disturbing you, in no particular order. Just notice what comes up as you search the whole episode from the original event until today, and stop at what is still disturbing you, and we will use it as a target for EMDR processing."*

Use continuous BLS during the G-Search.

Administer the Impact of Events Scale-R (IES-R) again. Check the SUD and use the IES-R once again after 3 months.

Comments about the process:

_____
_____
_____
_____

SUMMARY SHEET: The Recent Traumatic Episode Protocol (R-TEP): An Integrative Protocol for Early EMDR Intervention (EEI)

3A

Elan Shapiro and Brurit Laub
SUMMARY SHEET BY MARILYN LUBER

Name: _____ Day Today: _____
Date of Trauma: _____ Recent Trauma Episode: _____

☑ Check when task is completed, response has changed, or to indicate symptoms.

Note: This material is meant as a checklist for your response. Please keep in mind that it is only a reminder of different tasks that may or may not apply to your incident.

History Taking/Intake: Assessing Readiness for EEI

Phase 1: Client History—Focus on past traumas and resources

Administer the Impact of Event Scale (IES-R) questionnaire. Score:

Summarize Readiness: Severity, Motivation and Strengths (SMS) Rating

S	= Severity	(low)	1	2	3	4	5 (high)
M	= Motivation	(low)	1	2	3	4	5 (high)
S	= Strengths	(low)	1	2	3	4	5 (high)

(If Severity is high, minimum Motivation and Strengths should be 3 or higher)

Preparation/Resources

Phase 2: Preparation

Four Elements Exercise for Stress Management: ☐ Completed

Resource Connection: ☐ Completed

Other Self-Calming/Stabilization Exercises: _____
_____

Explanation of R-TEP: ☐ Completed
Episode Narrative: (main facts, no need to write all the details) _____

Continue On additional pages if needed.

Assessment and Desensitization: Points of Disturbance (PoDs)

Google Search for PoD #1 of T-Episode:

Summary Sheet: The Recent Traumatic Episode Protocol (R-TEP)

Phase 3: Assessment

(Do the full assessment, if possible. If high activation/inappropriate, do partial assessment.)

PoD#1: _____

NC: _____

PC: _____ VoC: _____ /7

Emotions: _____ SUD: _____ /10

Body Location: _____

Phase 4: Desensitization/Telescopic Processing

Main Strategy: EMDr Strategy

1. *EMDr Strategy* = when associations directly related to the current Traumatic Episode/ or are adaptive, continue with sets of BLS (or after two to three adaptive associations go back to PoD#1 and check SUD___/10).
   When associations do not relate to T-Episode, go BTT (PoD#1), check SUD _/10.
   When SUD reduces to ecological level go, to Installation.

If the PoD is an intrusion (intrusive image/sensation/feeling/thought), use EMD Strategy:

2. *EMD Strategy* = if associations are directly related to the PoD#1/adaptive, continue BLS. If associations do not relate to the PoD#1, go Back To Target (BTT) and check SUD _/10.

Note: If SUD does not reduce after about six to eight sets, "zoom out" in a natural transition to the EMDr Strategy.

When SUD does reduce to ecological level, go to Installation.

Google Search for PoD #2 of T-Episode: _____

_____

_____

_____

_____

Phase 3: Assessment

(Do the full assessment, if possible. If high activation/inappropriate, do partial assessment).

PoD#2: _____

NC: _____

PC: _____ VoC: _____ /7

_____ Emotions _____ SUD: _____ /10

Body Location: _____

Phase 4: Desensitization/Telescopic Processing

Main Strategy: EMDr Strategy

1. *EMDr Strategy* = when associations directly related to the current Traumatic Episode/ or are adaptive, continue with sets of BLS (or after two or three adaptive associations go back to PoD#2 and check SUD___/10).
   When associations do not relate to T-Episode, go BTT (PoD#2), check SUD _/10.
   When SUD reduces to ecological level, go to Installation.

2. *EMD Strategy* = if associations are directly related to the PoD#2___/adaptive, continue BLS.
   If associations do not relate to the PoD#2, go Back To Target (BTT) and check SUD _/10.

Note: If SUD does not reduce after about six to eight sets, "zoom out" in a natural transition to the EMDr Strategy.

When SUD does reduce to ecological level, go to Installation.

Google Search for PoD #3 of T-Episode: _____

_____

_____

_____

_____

Phase 3: Assessment

(Do the full assessment, if possible. If high activation/inappropriate, do partial assessment.)

PoD#3: _____

NC: _____

PC: _____ VoC: _____ /7

Emotions: _____ SUD: _____ /10

Phase 4: Desensitization/Telescopic Processing

Main Strategy: EMDR Strategy

1. *EMDr Strategy* = when associations directly related to the current Traumatic Episode/ or are adaptive, continue with sets of BLS (or after two or three adaptive associations go back to PoD#3 and check SUD___/10).
   When associations do not relate to T-Episode, go BTT (PoD#3), check SUD___/10.
   When SUD reduces to ecological level, go to Installation.

2. *EMD Strategy* = if associations are directly related to the PoD#3/adaptive, continue BLS. If associations do not relate to the PoD#3, go Back To Target (BTT) and check SUD___/10.

Note: If SUD does not reduce after about six to eight sets. "zoom out" in a natural transition to the EMDr Strategy.

When SUD does reduce to ecological level, go to Installation.

Google Search for PoD #___of T-Episode:

_____

_____

_____

_____

Phase 3: Assessment

(Do the full assessment, if possible. If high activation/inappropriate, do partial assessment).

PoD#3: _____

NC: _____

PC: _____ VoC: _____ /7

Emotions: _____ SUD: _____ /10

Phase 4: Desensitization/Telescopic Processing

Main Strategy: EMDr Strategy

1. *EMDr Strategy* = when associations directly related to the current Traumatic Episode/ or are adaptive, continue with sets of BLS (or after two or three adaptive associations go back to PoD#___ and check SUD___/10).
   When associations do not relate to T-Episode, go BTT (PoD#___), check SUD _/10.
   When SUD reduces to ecological level, go to Installation.

2. *EMD Strategy* = if associations are directly related to the PoD#_/adaptive, continue BLS. If associations do not relate to the PoD#_, go Back To Target (BTT) and check

Note: If SUD does not reduce after about six to eight sets, "zoom out" in a natural transition to the EMDr Strategy.

When SUD does reduce to ecological level, go to Installation.

Summary Sheet: The Recent Traumatic Episode Protocol (R-TEP) 57

Note: Make a strong closure at the end of each session, using the Four Elements Exercise for Stress Management, Closing Resource, etc.

Episode Level

When there are no more PoDs identified with the Google Search to process, check Episode SUD (E-SUD).

E-SUD: ____/10

When the SUD is ecological or can be viewed calmly, install Episode PC (E-PC).

Ask: *"What have you learned from this episode?"*

_____

_____

E-PC: _____

VoC: _____ /7

Phase 6: Episode Body Scan

Unresolved tension/tightness/unusual sensation: _____

_____

If SUD is still not ecological and the T-Episode cannot be viewed calmly, consider using the EMDR Standard Protocol for underlying issues beyond the T-Episode.

Client gives consent to new contract.   ☐ Completed

Phase 7: Closure of the Episode

IES-R is administered post session   ☐ Completed

Phase 8: Follow Up

Episode SUD:_/10

Resolved.   ☐ Completed

If SUD is not ecological, use G-Search to identify any residual targets.

_____

_____

3-month follow up: IES-R is implemented 3rd time: _____   ☐ Completed

Comments: _____

_____

_____

_____

_____

The EMDR Protocol for Recent Critical Incidents (EMDR-PRECI)

Ignacio Jarero and Lucina Artigas

Introduction

The EMDR Protocol for Recent Critical Incidents (EMDR-PRECI) is based on Dr. Shapiro's (2001) Recent Traumatic Events Protocol and the observations of Ignacio Jarero and Lucina Artigas during their many years of experience working in the field with natural or human provoked disaster survivors in Latin America and the Caribbean. In order to facilitate EMDR clinicians' use of this protocol, Drs. Marilyn Luber and Ignacio Jarero created this scripted version below.

EMDR-PRECI was developed in the field originally to treat clients after critical incidents (e.g., earthquake, flooding, landslides), where related stressful events continue for an extended period of time (often more than six months). Although it is a modification of Francine Shapiro's Recent Traumatic Events Protocol, it is also different in several important ways in order to accommodate the extended time frame with its continuum of stressful events, often along the themes of safety, responsibility, and choice. For Jarero and Uribe (2011, 2012) acute trauma situations are not only related to a time frame (e.g., days or months) but also to a post-trauma safety period.

Often, as a result of this ongoing lack of safety, the consolidation in memory of the original critical incident is prevented. The continuum of stressful events with similar emotions, somatic, sensory, and cognitive information does not give the state dependent traumatic memory sufficient time to consolidate into an integrated whole. Thus, the memory network remains in a permanent excitatory state, expanding with each subsequent stressful event in this continuum, like the ripple effect of a pebble thrown into a pond with the risk of PTSD and comorbid disorders growing with the number of exposures.

There is preliminary evidence supporting the efficacy of EMDR-PRECI in reducing symptoms of posttraumatic stress in adults and maintaining those effects despite ongoing threat and danger after a 7.2 earthquake in North Baja California and Mexico in 2010. This was part of a Disaster Mental Health Continuum of Care response (Jarero, Artigas, & Luber, 2011). The EMDR-PRECI was used in a human massacre situation with traumatized First Responders who were continuing to work under this extreme stress. They reported a reduction in self-report measures of posttraumatic stress and PTSD symptoms, resulting in the prevention of further development of chronic PTSD, and also included the increase in mechanisms of psychological and emotional resilience (Jarero & Uribe, 2011, 2012).

Clinical observations of the EMDR-PRECI during the reprocessing phases using the Standard EMDR Protocol's free associative processing showed that adjusting the EM length of sets and speed to the client's necessities, or using the Butterfly Hug as an alternative Bilateral Stimulation (BLS), resulted in a rapid progression of traumatic information processing in the perceptual, experiential, and meaning levels (Jarero & Uribe, 2011).

The EMDR Protocol for Recent Critical Incidents Script Notes

Benefits of the EMDR-PRECI

Some of the EMDR-PRECI benefits include the following:

- Transportability.
- Ease of use for both new and experienced EMDR practitioners.
- Time effectiveness—only one session was needed to achieve resolution of posttraumatic symptoms (Jarero & Uribe, 2011).
- No homework, thus facilitating a short duration of work in the field.
- Cross-cultural effectiveness for ongoing recent trauma, similar to the Standard EMDR Protocol's effectiveness for PTSD (Maxfield, 2008, 2009).

Core Concepts of EMDR-PRECI

Phase 1: Client History

- Narrative of the critical incident from right before the event occurred until the present moment, instead of just the narrative of the incident, unless the client is in great distress.
- Asking for the whole narrative instead of probing for the most disturbing aspect of the episode or early Client History.
- No bilateral stimulation (BLS) during the narrative to prevent processing.
- Administration of a scale before reprocessing to have a baseline measure and post-treatment measure to assess effectiveness.

Phase 2: Preparation

- Empowering the client through the use of self-administered BLS as in the Butterfly Hug.
- Self-soothing techniques such as Abdominal Breathing, the Concentration Exercise, and/or Pleasant Memory Technique that are easy to learn and promote self-efficacy.

Phase 3: Assessment

- Asking the client to *"Mentally run the movie of the whole episode from right before the beginning until today and at the end please let me know the worst part."* This instruction allows the identification of the worst part of the critical incident that then becomes the first target for reprocessing, once the client has containment and safety measures in place.
- If the client cannot think of a Negative Cognition (NC), the clinician can offer, "I am in danger."
- A Positive Cognition (PC) and Validity of Cognition (VoC) are not elicited here for a fragment—due to the continuum of stressful events—it makes it difficult for clients to find a PC for each fragment and may increase a sense of failure.

Phase 4: Desensitization

- During this phase, desensitize each separate aspect of the event and do not include the Installation Phase.
- Ask the client to visualize the entire sequence of the event again with eyes closed and reprocess *only fragments with disturbance*. Suggesting chronological order is simply a way to ensure that everything is processed. Depending on the circumstances (such as if there are many fragments for each client and few clinicians), the clinician can ask the client to visualize the entire sequence of the event with eyes closed and reprocess only fragments with disturbance.
- Do minimal intervention during the reprocessing phases to allow for the brain's natural processing.

- To maintain the clients in their window of tolerance, adjust the EM length of sets and speed to reflect the needs of the client.
- Use the Butterfly Hug as an alternative BLS.

Phase 5: Global Installation Phase

- Ask for a representative PC of the extended event.
- Check with the VoC.
- Link the PC and the entire event and add BLS.
- Keep doing BLS while information (disturbing or positive) is moving.
- When information stops moving, check VoC until the PC is fully installed (VoC = 7).

Supplement Step

- Close eyes, think of the PC, and review the whole sequence while continuing to hold the PC without BLS. If there are fragments that the PC feels less true, target that, using BLS.

Phase 6: Body Scan

- According to the EMDR Standard Protocol

Phase 7: Closure

- According to the EMDR Standard Protocol

Three-Pronged Approach

- According to the EMDR Standard Protocol

Post-Traumatic Growth

Administration of Instruments

The EMDR Protocol for Recent Critical Incidents Script

Phase 1: Client History

The clinician asks the client to describe the event in a narrative form from right before the event occurred until the present moment. If the client is in great distress (e.g., crying and not able to speak) or has physical complaints (e.g., headache, dizziness, nauseas, etc.) do not push for the narrative.

Say, "*Just give me a brief description of what happened.*"

_____

_____

Identify a series of separated aspects of the event (fragments).

Say, "*Without details, please tell me about the different aspects of what happened to you that are standing out for you.* "

1. _____
2. _____
3. _____
4. _____
5. _____

Note: Do not ask or probe for early client history, the most disturbing aspects of the event or do BLS during this phase.

At this point administer a scale/s (e.g., IES, IES-R, etc.) pre-reprocessing to have a baseline measure.

Phase 2: Preparation

Screen the Client to Make Sure He Is an Appropriate Candidate for the EMDR-PRECI

Does the client exhibit:

Life-threatening substance abuse:	☐ Yes	☐ No
Serious suicide attempts:	☐ Yes	☐ No
Self-mutilation:	☐ Yes	☐ No
Serious assaultive behavior:	☐ Yes	☐ No
Signs of dissociative disorders:	☐ Yes	☐ No*

*__Note:__ Peritraumatic dissociation or post-incident dissociative symptoms would be expected after critical incidents and are not considered a dissociative disorder.

Educate the Client About EMDR-AIP

> Say, *"When a disturbing event occurs, it can get locked in the brain with the original picture, sounds, thoughts, feelings, and body sensations. EMDR seems to stimulate the information and allows the brain to reprocess the experience. It is your own brain that will be doing the healing and you are the one in control. Do you accept treatment?"*

Instruct the client in the mechanics of EMDR such as the sitting position, distance, eye movement (EM), and the Butterfly Hug (BH). Eye movements are the first option for BLS. Use the Butterfly Hug (BH) as an alternative BLS. It is thought that the self-control obtained by clients using the BH may be an empowering factor that aids in their sense of safety while processing traumatic memories (Artigas & Jarero, 2009).

> Say, *"Now, remember, it is your own brain that is doing the healing and you are the one in control. I will ask you to mentally focus on the target and to follow my fingers (or any other BLS you are using)."*

Instruct the client in the metaphor (train) and stop signal/keep going signal.

> Say, *"In order to help you 'just notice' the experience, imagine riding on a train and the feelings, thoughts, etc., are just the scenery going by. Just let whatever happens, happen, and we will talk at the end of the set. Just tell me what comes up, and don't discard anything as unimportant. Any new information that comes to mind is connected in some way. If you want to stop, just raise your hand."*

The Butterfly Hug and Self-Soothing Exercises

THE BUTTERFLY HUG

> Say, *"Please watch me and do what I am doing. Cross your arms over your chest, so that the tip of the middle finger from each hand is placed below the clavicle or the collarbone, and the other fingers and hands cover the area that is located under the connection between the collarbone and the shoulder and the collarbone and sternum or breastbone. Hands and fingers must be as*

vertical as possible so that the fingers point toward the neck and not toward the arms.

Now interlock your thumbs to form the butterfly's body and the extension of your other fingers outward will form the butterfly's wings.
Your eyes can be closed, or partially closed, looking toward the tip of your nose. Next, you alternate the movement of your hands, like the flapping wings of a butterfly. Let your hands move freely. You can breathe slowly and deeply (abdominal breathing) *while you observe what is going through your mind and body such as thoughts, images, sounds, odors, feelings, and physical sensations without changing, pushing your thoughts away, or judging. You can pretend as though what you are observing is like clouds passing by."*

Instruct the client in the metaphor (train) and stop signal/keep going signal.

Say, *"In order to help you 'just notice' the experience, imagine riding on a train and the feelings, thoughts, etc. are just the scenery going by. If you need to stop during processing, you can hold up your hand as a signal, or turn your head."*

Teach the client self-soothing strategies such as Abdominal Breathing, Concentration Exercise, and the Pleasant Memory Technique.

ABDOMINAL BREATHING

Say, *"Close your eyes put one hand on your stomach and imagine that you have a balloon inside your stomach. Now, inhale and see how the balloon grows and moves your hand up. Now you can exhale and see how the balloon deflates and your hand goes down. Put all your attention in that. If anything distracts you gently return to the exercise."*

Do this exercise for 5 minutes.

CONCENTRATION EXERCISE (5 MINUTES)

Say, *"I would like you to take a little time to think about your breathing. Notice when you are inhaling and say to yourself, 'I am inhaling,' and then notice when you are exhaling and say to yourself, 'I am exhaling.' Continue to allow your attention to focus on your breath, for a while longer, gently bringing yourself back—if you are distracted—to the inhaling and exhaling of your breath."*

Do this exercise for 5 minutes.

PLEASANT MEMORY

Say, *"Remember a time when you were calm or happy. (Pause). Now, put your hand on your chest and let those good feelings and positive physical sensations expand throughout your body. Good. Continue to allow your attention to focus on these good feelings and sensations for a while longer, gently bringing yourself back—if you are distracted—to the happy and calm feelings you are feeling."*
At the end, say, *"As you open your eyes, remember that in the future all you have to do to bring back the memory is to place your hand over the center of your chest."*

Do this exercise for 5 minutes.

Phase 3: Assessment

Run the movie to establish the first target.

> Say, *"Mentally run the movie of the whole event from right before the beginning until today and at the end please let me know the worst part, the worst fragment."*

_____
_____

Note: Access the fragment Image, Negative Cognition, Emotion, SUDs, and Location of Physical sensation. DO NOT ASK FOR THE PC OR VoC.

Picture

> Say, *"What picture represents the most disturbing aspect or moment of that part or fragment?"*

_____
_____

If there are many choices or if the client becomes confused, the clinician assists by asking the following:

> Say, *"What picture represents the most traumatic moment of the event?"*

_____
_____

When a picture is unavailable, the clinician merely invites the client to do the following:

> Say, *"Think of the most disturbing aspect or moment of that part or fragment."*

_____

Negative Cognition (NC)

> Say, *"What words best go with the picture that express your negative belief about yourself now?"*

_____

Note: The clinician only offers an NC such as, "I'm in danger," if clients are unable to come up with their own NC.

Emotions

> Say, *"When you bring up the picture* (or disturbing aspect/moment) *and those words* _____ (clinician states the negative cognition), *what emotion do you feel now?"*

_____

Subjective Units of Disturbance (SUD)

> Say, *"On a scale of 0 to 10, where 0 is no disturbance or neutral and 10 is the highest disturbance you can imagine, how disturbing does it feel now?"*

> 0   1   2   3   4   5   6   7   8   9   10
> (no disturbance)   (highest disturbance)

Location of Body Sensation

Say, *"Where do you feel it* (the disturbance) *in your body?"*

___

Continue with Phase 4: Desensitization Phase.

Phase 4: Desensitization Phase/Reprocessing

Target and Reprocess in the Following Sequence:

a. Elicit worst fragment (see above).
b. After you have processed the worst fragment always elicit other fragments using the run the movie procedure (see below). Assess and reprocess individually only fragments/parts with disturbance using Phases 3 and 4.

Run the Movie

Have the client visualize and fully experience the entire sequence with eyes closed from right before the beginning until today and then ask for any other part that is disturbing. Client should have full association with the material while running the movie. If there is disturbance, the client should inform the clinician at the end of the movie.

Say, *"Close your eyes, and mentally run the movie of the whole event from right before the beginning until today making sure to really allow yourself to feel every part of the experience, and at the end please let me know any other part that disturbs you now."*

___

___

Reprocess only fragments/parts with disturbance following Phases 3 and 4. At this point, it is not necessary to reprocess each fragment with the full Standard EMDR Protocol (meaning Phases 5 and 6) because we are not working with a consolidated memory network.

This procedure is repeated until the entire event can be visualized from start to finish without emotional, cognitive, or somatic distress.

Note: Access the fragment Image, Negative Cognition, Emotion, SUDs, and Location of Physical sensation. DO NOT ASK FOR THE PC OR VoC.

Picture

Say, *"What picture represents the most disturbing aspect or moment of that part or fragment?"*

___

___

If there are many choices or if the client becomes confused, the clinician assists by asking the following:

Say, *"What picture represents the most traumatic moment of the event?"*

___

___

When a picture is unavailable, the clinician merely invites the client to do the following:

Say, *"Think of the most disturbing aspect or moment of that part or fragment."*

___

Negative Cognition (NC)

Say, "*What words best go with the picture that express your negative belief about yourself now?*"

___

Note: The clinician only offers an NC such as, "I'm in danger," if clients are unable to come up with their own NC.

Emotions

Say, "*When you bring up the picture* (or disturbing aspect/moment) *and those words* _____ (clinician states the negative cognition), *what emotion do you feel now?*"

___

Subjective Units of Disturbance (SUD)

Say, "*On a scale of 0 to 10, where 0 is no disturbance or neutral and 10 is the highest disturbance you can imagine, how disturbing does it feel now?*"

0   1   2   3   4   5   6   7   8   9   10
(no disturbance)   (highest disturbance)

Location of Body Sensation

Say, "*Where do you feel it* (the disturbance) *in your body?*"

___

Phase 4: Desensitization

Continue with Phase 4: Desensitization Phase. Also see Phase 3 above.

Phase 5: Global Installation Phase

When the entire event can be visualized from start to finish without emotional, cognitive, or somatic distress, elicit the representative Positive Cognition for the *entire* event.

Say, "*When you bring up the entire incident, what would you like to believe about yourself now?*"

___

Check the VoC.

Say, "*Think about the whole incident. How true do those words* _____ (clinician repeats the positive cognition) *feel to you now on a scale of 1 to 7, where 1 feels completely false and 7 feels completely true?*"

1   2   3   4   5   6   7
(completely false)   (completely true)

Link the PC and the entire event and add BLS.

Say, "*Think of the entire event* (or incident) *and hold it together with the words* _____ (repeat the selected positive cognition), *now let whatever happens, happen.*"

If necessary, tell the client that the PC and the event are linked together, only at the beginning, but not during BLS.

Do sets of BLS (same speed and approximate duration as in the Desensitization Phase) to fully install the PC (VoC = 7).

At the end of the set say, *"Take a breath ... what do you notice now?"*
If disturbing material arises say, *"Go with that"* or *"Notice that."*
Keep doing BLS while information (disturbing or positive) is moving.
When information stops moving, check the VoC until the PC is fully installed (VoC = 7).

Say, *"When you think of the entire event, how true do those words _____ (clinician repeats the positive cognition) feel to you now on a scale of 1 to 7, where 1 feels completely false and 7 feels completely true?"*

1   2   3   4   5   6   7
(completely false)   (completely true)

If VoC < 7, check for a Blocking Belief.

Say, *"What prevents this from being a 7?"*

_____
_____

Reprocess with BLS whatever the client reports until the VoC = 7.

Supplemental Step (F. Shapiro, 2010, Personal Communication)

Say, *"Close your eyes, think of the positive cognition, and review the whole sequence in your mind as you are holding the PC."*

On completion, say, *"Does the positive cognition feel less than true on any part/fragment of the sequence?"*

_____

If so, target that part with BLS.

If there is disturbance, say, *"Continue reprocessing until the disturbance clears. Let me know when that occurs."*

_____

This procedure is repeated until the entire event can be visualized from start to finish with the PC, without emotional, cognitive, or somatic distress.

Phase 6: Body Scan

Run a Body Scan following the Standard EMDR Procedure. Reprocess any disturbance or enhance positive affect or body sensations with BLS (with 25–30 sets of BLS).

Say, *"Close your eyes and keep in mind the entire event and the _____ (repeat the positive cognition). Then bring your attention to the different parts of your body, starting with your head and working downward. Any place you find tension, tightness, or unusual sensation, tell me."*

_____

If there is disturbance, say, *"Continue reprocessing until the disturbance clears. Let me know when that occurs."*

_____

This procedure is repeated until the Body Scan is clear.

Phase 7: Closure

Use the Standard EMDR Protocol to close the session.

> Say, *"We are almost out of time and we will need to stop soon. You have done some very good work and I appreciate the effort you have made. How are you feeling?"*

_____
_____

> Say, *"Processing may continue after our session. You may or may not notice new insights, thoughts, memories, physical sensations, or dreams. Please make a note of whatever you notice. We will talk about that at our next session. Remember to use one of the self-soothing strategies as needed, or use the Butterfly Hug, to desensitize any highly disturbing affect that arise if self-soothing techniques were not effective quickly enough."*

Three-Pronged Approach

1. Past memories: the traumatic incident memories already reprocessed.
2. Present Triggers: Reprocess present triggers with the client. Each trigger may be connected to different situations that need different skill sets or information to optimize future functioning.
3. Future Template.

Present Triggers

Reprocess *present stimuli* that may cause a startle response, nightmares, and other reminders of the event that the client still finds disturbing, if necessary.

> Say, *"Are you having any other triggers to situations, events, or stimuli that are related to this event?"*

List of Situations and Events That Trigger the Critical Incident

_____
_____
_____

Picture

> Say, *"What picture represents the disturbing aspect or moment of the event?"*

_____
_____

If there are many choices or if the client becomes confused, the clinician assists by asking the following:

> Say, *"What picture represents the most traumatic moment of the event?"*

_____
_____

When a picture is unavailable, the clinician merely invites the client to do the following:

Say, *"Think of the disturbing aspect or moment of the event.*

_____

_____

Negative Cognition (NC)

Say, *"What words best go with the picture that express your negative belief about yourself now?"*

_____

_____

Subjective Units of Disturbance (SUD)

Say, *"On a scale of 0 to 10, where 0 is no disturbance or neutral and 10 is the highest disturbance you can imagine, how disturbing does it feel now?"*

 0   1   2   3   4   5   6   7   8   9   10
(no disturbance)   (highest disturbance)

Location of Body Sensation

Say, *"Where do you feel it* (the disturbance) *in your body?"*

_____

_____

Continue with Phases 4 through 7 for the situation, event, or stimulus that triggers you from above and any others. After processing the first triggered situation, check to see if any of the others mentioned are still active; if not, proceed to the next question. If there are more triggers that need to be processed, go ahead and reprocess that experience.

Future Template

The clinician asks the client to run a movie of the desired response to cope in the future.

Say, *"This time, I'd like you to close your eyes and play a movie, imagining yourself coping effectively with _____ (state where client will be) in the future. With the new positive belief _____ (state positive belief) and your new sense of _____ (strength, clarity, confidence, calm), imagine stepping into the future. Imagine yourself coping with ANY challenges that come your way. Make sure that this movie has a beginning, middle, and end. Notice what you are seeing, thinking, feeling, and experiencing in your body. Let me know if you hit any blocks. If you do, just open your eyes and let me know. If you don't hit any blocks, let me know when you have viewed the whole movie."*

_____

_____

If the client hits blocks, address as above with BLS until the disturbance dissipates.

Say, *"Go with that."*

Post-Traumatic Growth

Post-traumatic growth is positive change experienced as the result of the struggle with a major life crisis or a traumatic event. At the end, ask the participant for the positive learning they have gained from the experience.

Say, *"Is there any new positive learning or change you have had as a result of this experience?"*

_____

_____

Administration of Instruments

Use the instruments that are relevant to the work that you are doing in your country. In Mexico, the instruments are the following: Short PTSD Rating Interview (SPRINT) (Connor & Davidson, 2001) and Impact of Event Scale-Revised (IES-R) (Weiss & Marmar, 1997).

Say, *"Please fill in these questionnaires."*

Jarero and Artigas suggest that the EMDR-PRECI must be part of a community based trauma response program that provides a continuum of care for the treatment and management of individual and group reactions to shared traumatic events. This continuum of care must be accessible to the community members and sensitive to each participant's gender, developmental stage, ethno-cultural background, and magnitude of trauma exposure (Macy et al., 2004).

SUMMARY SHEET:
The EMDR Protocol for Recent Critical Incidents (EMDR-PRECI)

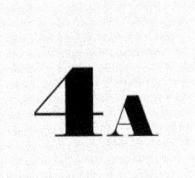

Ignacio Jarero and Lucina Artigas
SUMMARY SHEET BY MARILYN LUBER

Name: _____ Diagnosis: _____

☑ Check when task is completed, response has changed, or to indicate symptoms.

Phase 1: Client History

Event Date: _____

Event Narrative From Before the Event to the Present Moment: _____
_____
_____
_____
_____
_____
_____

Different Aspects that Stand Out:

1. _____
2. _____
3. _____
4. _____
5. _____

Phase 2: Preparation

Screening:

Life-threatening substance abuse	☐ Yes	☐ No
Serious suicide attempts:	☐ Yes	☐ No
Self-mutilation:	☐ Yes	☐ No
Serious assaultive behavior:	☐ Yes	☐ No
Signs of dissociative disorders	☐ Yes	☐ No

Educate about EMDR: ☐ Completed

BLS: EMS _____ Sound _____ Tapping _____ Butterfly Hug _____

For Adults Add: Abdominal Breathing _____ Concentration Exercise _____
Pleasant Memory _____

Instruments Administered Pre EMDR-PRECIS: ☐ Completed

_____
_____
_____

Phase 3: Assessment

Run the Movie of the Whole Episode From Beginning Until Today—Worst Part: _____
_____
_____

Picture

NC: _____

Emotions: _____

SUDs: _____/10

Location: _____

Phase 4: Desensitization

Elicit Other Fragments and Run the Movie

TARGET AND REPROCESS THE WORST FRAGMENT—SEE ABOVE

1. _____
2. _____
3. _____
4. _____
5. _____

Picture

NC: _____

Emotions: _____

SUDs: _____/10

Location: _____

Run the Movie—Eyes Closed. Disturbances:

1. _____
2. _____
3. _____
4. _____
5. _____

Phase 5: Global Installation Phase

PC for Entire Incident: _____

VoC: _____/7

Link PC + Target + BLS

_____

_____

Check VoC until VoC = 7/7

VoC: _____/7

Supplemental Step

Close eyes + PC + Review the whole sequence

PC: _____True _____Less True

If less true, target part less true.

_____

_____

Phase 6: Body Scan

Any issues? _____

_____

If so, target until decreased.

Phase 7: Closure—Standard

Three-Pronged Approach

1. Past memories already processed
2. Present trigger
3. Future template

Present Triggers

Situations and Events Triggering the Incident

1. _____
2. _____
3. _____
4. _____
5. _____

   Picture: _____

   NC: _____

   PC: _____

   VoC: _____/7

   Emotions: _____

   SUDs: _____/10

   Location: _____

Future Template

Run the Movie

Where: _____

PC: _____

Positive Attribute: _____

Blocks:

1. _____
2. _____
3. _____
4. _____
5. _____

Post-Traumatic Growth

_____

_____

Instruments Administered Post EMDR-PRECI:

_____

_____

_____

EMDR Early Intervention for Groups

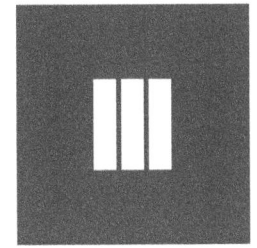

Inspiration to work in groups began at the House of Culture in Acapulco in 1997, after Hurricane Pauline ravaged the west coast of Mexico. Ignacio "Nacho" Jarero, Lucy Artigas, Teresa Lopez Cano, and the three Judys (Albert, Boel, and Jones) wanted to help respond to the disaster. They were shocked to find 200 survivors on their doorstep when they arrived and had to think quickly and figure out what they could do. When Lucy saw what an effort the women and children made to come and get help, she realized that this would be their only chance to make a difference. She was inspired then—having attended an EMDR Training—and said, "Put your hand on your chest and put the other hand on the other side of your chest, and just tap back and forth." At that moment, the Butterfly Hug was born. For 15 days, this team worked to support and assist those suffering in the aftermath of the hurricane.

One week later, the true start of the early group intervention began when four team members went in search of a school whose teachers and pupils needed assistance. The school was flooded and the children and teachers were sitting under a mango tree. They began their intervention right away. Because there were no pencils, crayons, or paper, Lucy had the children think about the worst part of the hurricane and draw it in the sand with their fingers; then, they did the Butterfly Hug. Afterwards, they erased the picture with their fingers and drew the next picture that came to mind; they did this three or four times until the fear and bad memories disappeared. Through Lucy's creativity and the help of the team, the EMDR Integrative Group Treatment Protocol (IGTP) was created. Later, when they got supplies, the children used paper and crayons for their pictures.

Before the team's eyes, they saw the process of EMDR unfold. The children showed their distress and terror first and then as they developed their drawings, the pain and suffering decreased until the children said that the pictures were done and they wanted to go out and play. Teresa supported their natural movement with more bilateral stimulation and asked them to march. The children's release from their trauma was so rapid that Nacho thought, "It was magic in front of our eyes!" This was the moment that Nacho and Lucy's lives changed forever—as did all of those survivors of devastating trauma who now would have the gift of the IGTP. The beginning of the IGTP's healing voyage around the world had begun.

After they beheld "the miracle," Lucy, Nacho, Nicté, and Teresa refined these ideas further. Over the next 10 years, as a part of their disaster response, they gathered data, took pictures, and made films until the protocol evolved into the actual EMDR-IGTP. By 1998, they founded the Mexican Association for Mental Health in Crisis (AMAMECRISIS), a nonprofit private organization whose members are mental health professionals trained in the prevention and treatment of traumatic stress, providing services in Mexico, Europe, and Central and South America (Luber, 2010, April).

The following story, taken from *Eye Movement Desensitization and Reprocessing (EMDR) Scripted Protocols: Basics and Special Situations* (Luber, 2009a, pp. 277–278), tells the wide-ranging consequences of Lucy's inspiration:

At a recent conference on EMDR, my colleague, Gary Quinn, expressed a wish to meet the creators of the EMDR Integrative Group Protocol (IGTP). As luck would have it, I happened to know where they were and I introduced Gary to Lucy Artigas and Ignacio Jarero, two of the four originators of the IGTP. The reason Gary wanted to meet them was to thank them for the tremendous contributions that they have made to the world of trauma treatment, and he went on to tell them several stories about the uses of the IGTP in four different countries.

The first began in a country that had suffered from a devastating earthquake. A colleague of Gary's had gone there to help and used the IGTP. In the first city, he worked with 1,200 children who had lost both of their parents and he was amazed that—despite his not knowing the local dialects—he began to see in the children's drawings the changes in their perceptions concerning this devastating natural disaster. He also noted that their demeanors changed and their spirits rose. This colleague traveled to a number of cities, working in the same manner and with the same results.

A group had gathered around us as Gary continued talking to Lucy and Nacho and there was not a dry eye in the group.

Gary went on to tell them of his own experience in Israel after one of the recent wars that had children and their families sequestered in bomb shelters. As Gary used IGTP, he began to see the transformation of the children's experience, again, through their drawings. What started as terrible pictures of death and destruction, as the process progressed, turned into drawings that began to show grass and then people going about their daily living. At one point, when they were beginning to exit the shelter, the bombing began anew and a little girl began to cry. Gary reminded her of the Butterfly Hug (a method for self-bilateral stimulation created by Lucy); she began to do it, and immediately felt better. This was repeated with the same results in the other shelters that Gary and his colleagues worked.

In 2007, Gary went to the EMDR-European conference in Paris. There, he saw the work that a Palestinian colleague had done treating children with IGTP. Although there seemed to be a certain political influence in the first pictures, the children progressed in the same positive way—and appeared almost identical—to the pictures of the Israeli children. This was the same type of result that occurred when the IGTP was used with children in Thailand after the tsunami. Gary was astounded. At that moment, he felt transformed by the profound understanding of the universal nature of all peoples—no matter their culture or their political views—and how this extraordinary treatment has tapped into the common innate ability to heal.

Every day we are confronted with disasters that occur around the world. We are seeing an ever-increasing need to treat large groups of people, to assist them in returning to functioning adaptively as quickly as possible. In Artigas, Jarero, Alcalá, and López Cano's, "The EMDR Integrative Group Treatment Protocol (IGTP) for Children," and Jarero and Artigas's chapter, "The EMDR Integrative Group Treatment Protocol (IGTP) for Adults," along with their Summary Sheets, we find ways to work with large groups of children and/or adults under the worst of circumstances.

All of these chapters include separate summary sheets for the child/participant and the adult/clinician/leader to assist in data entry and a tickler reminding clinicians about the elements of these protocols.

The IGTP and the work inspired by it has been critical to the healing of people around the world. In 2007, Luci Artigas and Ignacio Jarero received the Francine Shapiro Award from EMDR Ibero-America. Francine herself underlined the importance of their contribution:

And if others will follow in their footsteps, and conduct the randomized research needed to solidify the work in the eyes of the world, to have it declared "empirically validated" by the large international organizations such as UNICEF, then thousands and thousands more will be healed in the coming years. So as you applaud the work of these wonderful people, please see what a difference can be made through a dedication to relieve suffering. (Luber, 2009a, p. 278)

The concept behind this book has been in response to those mental health practitioners who have needed to gather together the protocols for recent trauma after a local or national disaster. It is clear that more and more clinicians are being trained and responding in their local environments, states, countries, and travelling elsewhere to assist colleagues in what seems an avalanche of man-made and natural disasters that are befalling us. Francine's request is being actualized as more and more clinicians are dedicating themselves to relieve suffering around the world and research is beginning to grow.

The EMDR Integrative Group Treatment Protocol (IGTP) for Children

Lucina Artigas, Ignacio Jarero, Nicté Alcalá, and Teresa López Cano

Introduction

The effectiveness of Eye Movement Desensitization and Reprocessing (EMDR) with trauma survivors has been widely reported (e.g., Gelinas, 2003; Ironson, Freund, Strauss, & Williams, 2002; Korn & Leeds, 2002; Lee, Gavriel, Drummond, Richards, & Greenwald, 2002; Manfield & Shapiro, 2003; McCullough, 2002; Perkins & Rouanzoin, 2002). Studies support the use of EMDR in the treatment of symptoms caused by trauma in children and adolescents (Cocco & Sharpe, 1993; Greenwald, 1994, 1998, 1999, 2000; Johnson, 1998; Lovett, 1999; Pellicer, 1993; Puffer, Greenwald, & Elrod, 1998; Russell & O'Connor, 2002; Scheck, Schaeffer, & Gillette, 1998; Shapiro, 1991; Soberman, Greenwald, & Rule, 2002; Stewart & Bramson, 2000; Taylor, 2002; Tinker & Wilson, 1999).

Studies have evaluated the usefulness of EMDR following disaster events (Fernandez, Gallinari, & Lorenzetti, 2004; Grainger, Levin, Allen-Byrd, Doctor, & Lee, 1997; Jarero, Artigas, & Hartung, 2006; Jarero, Artigas, & Montero, 2008; Konuk et al., 2006), finding that this approach could be effective in significantly reducing posttraumatic symptoms. EMDR has been reported as effective in the treatment of children following a hurricane in Hawaii (Chemtob, Nakashima, & Carlson, 2002), with victims of the 9/11 terrorist attacks in New York City (Silver, Rogers, Knipe, & Colelli, 2005), and with victims of earthquakes in Turkey (Korkmazlar-Oral & Pamuk, 2002).

Group therapy is a well-proven form of treatment for traumatized children and adolescents (Cemalovic, 1997; Kristal-Andersson, 2000; Meichenbaum, 1994; Samec, 2001).

The EMDR-Integrative Group Treatment Protocol (IGTP) Script Notes

The EMDR-IGTP was developed by members of AMAMECRISIS when they were overwhelmed by the extensive need for mental health services after Hurricane Pauline ravaged the western coast of Mexico in 1997. This protocol combines the Standard EMDR Treatment Phases 1 through 8 (Shapiro, 1995, 2001) with a Group Therapy model (Jarero, Artigas, Mauer, Lopez Cano, & Alcalá, 1999; Artigas, Jarero, Mauer, López Cano, & Alcalá, 2000). It is hypothesized that the resulting format offers a more extensive reach than individual EMDR applications and that the treatment may produce a more effective outcome than expected from traditional group therapy (Jarero et al., 2008).

Designed initially for work with children, the EMDR-IGTP has also been found suitable for group work with adults (Jarero, & Artigas, 2010). The protocol is structured within a play therapy format and has been used with disaster victims ages 7 to 50 + . Because of its utility, it has been used in the original format in multiple settings around the world (Aduriz, Knopfler, & Bluthgen, 2009; Errebo, Knipe, Forte, Karlin, & Altayli, 2008; Jarero et al., 2006, 2008), or with adaptations to meet the circumstances (Fernandez et al., 2004; Gelbach & Davis, 2007; Korkmazlar-Oral & Pamuk, 2002; Wilson, Tinker, Hofmann, Becker, & Marshall, 2000; Zaghrout-Hodali, Alissa, & Dodgson, 2008). "EMDR-IGTP has been found effective in several field trials and has been used for thousands of disaster survivors around the world" (Maxfield, 2008, p. 75). This protocol is also known as the Group Butterfly Hug Protocol, The EMDR Group Protocol for Children, and the Children's Group Protocol.

The protocol was designed to accomplish the following main objectives:

- Be part of a comprehensive program (continuum of care) for trauma treatment.
- Identify those who need further assistance.
- Reduce posttraumatic symptoms.
- Confront traumatic material.
- Bring to conscious awareness those aspects of the trauma that were dissociated.
- Facilitate the expression of painful emotions or shameful behaviors.
- Offer the patient support and empathy.
- Condense the different aspects of trauma into representative and more manageable images.
- Increase patient's perception of mastery over the distressing elements of the traumatic experience.
- Reprocess traumatic memories.
- Treat more clients for the same experience.
- Normalize the reactions: The clients can see that their reactions are normal since other patients are working on their memories in the same manner.

Advantages of this protocol are:

- Group treatment can be used in nonprivate settings such as under a mango tree, in shelters and open-air clinics, and so forth.
- Clients in the group do not have to verbalize information about the trauma.
- Therapy can be done on subsequent days, and there is no need for homework between sessions.
- Protocol is easily taught to both new and experienced EMDR practitioners.
- Equally effective cross-culturally.
- People are treated more quickly, involving larger segments of the affected community.
- When single clinicians are able to be assisted by paraprofessionals, teachers, or family members, it allows for a wider application of this protocol in societies with few mental health professionals.

The EMDR Integrative Group Treatment Protocol Script

Phase 1: Client History

First, team members educate teachers, parents, and relatives about the course of trauma and enlist these individuals to identify affected children. Team members have to be aware of the needs of the clients within their extended families, communities, and cultures.

Family members can be involved in a continuum of passive-to-active roles. The family member can be asked simply to be present and to witness or to perform a function as part of the Emotional Protection Team (EPT).

> Say, *"I would like to ask the team members if they could please help the children that need assistance in writing or in understanding anything that we will be doing today."*

Phase 2: Preparation—First Part

The professionals who work with survivors of a traumatic event, especially in the immediate aftermath of trauma, should listen actively and supportively, but not probe for details and emotional responses or push for more information than survivors are comfortable providing. Professionals must tread lightly in the wake of disaster so as not to disrupt natural social networks of healing and support. During this protocol, the rest of the team forms an EPT around the children in order to be aware of their emotional reactions and help them when necessary. We recommend a ratio of one team member for eight children. If you do not have enough clinicians in the team, the children's teachers and family members can help.

This phase begins with an integration exercise. At first, obtain the children's attention and establish rapport. We use a little Mexican doll called Lupita, a little drum, and a dolphin puppet, but any other materials may be used. It is helpful for the mental health professionals to use whatever techniques they prefer to capture the child's attention and establish rapport.

The aims are (a) to familiarize the children with the space where they are going to work or play, (b) to encourage the children to approach the therapist in order to establish rapport and trust, and (c) to facilitate group formation.

Lupita, the doll, introduces the drum and the dolphin to her friends. The therapist plays soft sounds on the drum and asks the children to approach as giants; when she plays loud sounds, they have to retreat as little people. The therapist may say something like the following:

> Say, *"Hi, my name is Lupita* (therapist holds the doll and shows the drum and the dolphin). *This is my drum and this is my dolphin and I want you to get to know them. As you listen to the sound of the drum, please become the largest giants you can be and come forward* (play soft sounds). *Wonderful. Now* (play loud sounds), *become little people and move away as fast as you can."*

During this time, the team leader says whatever she needs to say according to the circumstances. As this is creative work, the leader must have knowledge of children and how to work with them empathically in a group setting.

The therapist uses the dolphin to show the children different expressions of feeling. The therapist makes the dolphin form big and small mouths, mouths that look happy, sad, bored, afraid, surprised, angry, and so forth, and the children follow the leader by imitating the expressions of the dolphin.

> Say, *"Here is the dolphin and see how he makes his mouth soooo big and then soooo small. What does he look like now* (make a happy face)?"

___

> Say, *"Can you make your face look like the dolphin's happy face? Go ahead. That is great!"*

___

> Say, *"What does he look like now* (make a sad face)?

___

> Say, *"Can you make your face look like the dolphin's sad face? Go ahead. That is great!"*

___

> Say, *"What does he look like now* (make a scary face)?

___

Say, *"Can you make your face look like the dolphin's scary face? Go ahead. That is great!"*

Say, *"What does he look like now (make a surprised face)?"*

Say, *"Can you make your face look like the dolphin's surprised face? Go ahead. That is great!"*

Say, *"What does he look like now (make an angry face)?"*

Say, *"Can you make your face look like the dolphin's angry face? Go ahead. That is great!"*

Again, the team leader works with the group in the way that is particular to the group. The dolphin helps the children make contact with their emotions, expressing them through their bodies.

Using the doll, the team leader teaches the children the abdominal breathing technique.

Say, *"Close your eyes, put one hand on your stomach and imagine that you have a balloon inside your stomach. Now, inhale and see how the balloon grows and moves your hand up. Now you can exhale and see how the balloon deflates and your hand goes down. Just observe."*

The Butterfly Hug

The team leader teaches the children the Butterfly Hug (Artigas et al., 2000).

Say, *"Please watch me and do what I am doing. Cross your arms over your chest, so that the tip of the middle finger from each hand is placed below the clavicle or the collarbone, and the other fingers and hands cover the area that is located under the connection between the collarbone and the shoulder and the collarbone and sternum or breastbone. Hands and fingers must be as vertical as possible so that the fingers point toward the neck and not toward the arms. Now interlock your thumbs to form the butterfly's body and the extension of your other fingers outward will form the butterfly's wings.*
Your eyes can be closed, or partially closed, looking toward the tip of your nose. Next, you alternate the movement of your hands, like the flapping wings of a butterfly. Let your hands move freely. You can breathe slowly and deeply (abdominal breathing), *while you observe what is going through your mind and body such as thoughts, images, sounds, odors, feelings, and physical sensations without changing, pushing your thoughts away, or judging. You can pretend as though what you are observing is like clouds passing by."*

It is important to observe the children to make sure that they are able to follow along with you. If not, members of the EPT can be alert and quietly go up to a child to help as needed and then return to teaching the Butterfly Hug.

To install the safe or calm place:

Say, *"Now, please close your eyes and use your imagination to go to a place where you feel safe or calm. What images, colors, and sounds, for example, do you see in your safe place."*

After the answer, say, *"Please do the BH six to eight times while you concentrate on your safe or calm place."*

The EPT members are spaced around the group so that they are able to hear the children's answers. Sometimes, children will say their answers out loud, giving the members of the team the possibility of responding to each individual child as needed. It is important to observe the children to make sure that they are able to follow and find a safe/calm place that they have imagined. Members of the EPT can be alert and quietly go up to a child to help as needed.

The goal here is to make sure that the children have found a safe/calm place in their imagination.

Optional

Say, *"Now, please take out your paper and draw the safe/calm place that you imagined. When you are finished, please do the Butterfly Hug six to eight times while looking at your drawing."*

The children can take the picture home to use it with the Butterfly Hug whenever they need to feel better.

Say, *"You are welcome to take your picture home and you can use it with the Butterfly Hug whenever you need to feel better."*

The Butterfly Hug is used to anchor positive affect, cognitions, and physical sensations associated with images produced by the technique of "guided imagination."

Make sure to notice the children's responses, as there is no talking during the process so that the children are not taken out of their process. If a child is experiencing any difficulty, one of the EPT members can assist the child.

Trauma Work

Say, *"Please raise your hand if you have been having trouble sleeping, are scared, if you feel sad, if you still have nightmares, if you feel angry, or if you often think about and remember the natural or human-provoked disaster that you have suffered."*

The therapist goes on to say, *"It is normal for you to feel this way; you are normal boys and girls who have suffered an abnormal experience, and that is why it is normal for you to have these feelings. It is also normal to have different feelings than your friends and other children, since each person experiences and feels things differently. This is really normal."*

The aim is to validate the signs and symptoms of posttraumatic stress.

The therapist goes on and says, *"When you return home after this exercise, you can talk to the people you trust about your thoughts and feelings, as much as you want and when you feel most comfortable doing so."*

The aim is to verbalize the traumatic memories and to respond to the acute need that arises in many survivors to share their experience, while at the same time respecting their natural inclination with regard to how much, when, and to whom they talk.

CHILD'S REACTION TO TRAUMATIC EVENTS SCALE

The team administers the Child's Reaction to Traumatic Events Scale (CRTES) (Jones 1997; Jones, Fletcher, & Ribbe, 2004) here at the end of the first part of the Preparation phase.

Say, *"Here is a scale for you to look at. Please answer the questions on it. If you have any questions, please ask one of the Emotional Protection Team Members to help you out."*

Standardized psychological assessment is used cautiously. It is helpful for team members to be concerned about the rapport with the family members and children. They need to demonstrate by their behavior that they are truly interested in the children as human beings and not as objects of scientific curiosity. This custom weakens the scientific value of data gathered, while it respects the wishes of our Latin American clients not to be stigmatized by formal testing procedures. In our experience, clients also tend to reject assistance from those they judge to be opportunists, in this case anyone who seems interested in the victim as an object of study.

Phase 2: Preparation—Second Part

Show the children the faces that measure SUDs from 0 to 10, with 0 being no disturbance, and 10 being maximum disturbance. If you do not have the original faces you can draw them on the blackboard.

> Say, *"Here are faces that measure our feelings on a 0 to 10 scale, where 0 does not bother you at all, and 10 bothers you the most possible."*

Note: Clinicians are welcome to use the best words and pictures possible for their population.

> Familiarize the children with the scale.
>
> Say, *"How do you feel when you get good grades? Please point to the face that describes how you feel."*
> Now say, *"How do you feel when you are sick? Please point to the face that tells us how you feel."*

We have observed that the children who are not yet familiar with the numbers will sometimes say a number and point to a face that does not correspond. Thus, it is better to pick the face they point to over the number they say (one of the members of the EPT can write the correct number). The members of the EPT hand out white pieces of paper and crayons to each of the children (have extra crayons in case the children ask for more).

> Say, *"Please write your name and age on the top left side of the paper* (show how to do it)*."*
>
> EPT members can aid those who cannot do it.
>
> Say, *"Now, please divide the other side of the paper into four equal parts like this. Draw a cross at the center like this and write a small letter at the top left corner of each section like this."*
>
> The therapist shows them how to do it on the blackboard and the EPT helps.

Note: In this protocol we had to divide the sheet of paper in four, given the scarcity of the materials in the shelters, but it is acceptable to use four sheets of paper, making sure that each has the name and the age of the child and the corresponding letter, so that the sequence can be identified.

Phase 3: Assessment

The therapist says, *"Whoever remembers what happened during the event_____* (mention the event—hurricane, flooding, explosion, etc.), *please raise your hands."*

The children raise their hands.

> Say, *"Now, close your eyes and observe what makes you the most frightened, sad, or angry about that event_____* (mention the event) *NOW."*

The therapist continues, *"Take whatever emerges from your head to your neck, to your arms, to your hands and fingers, to the crayon, and now open your eyes and draw it in square A."*

When all the children are finished, show them the faces again.

Say, *"Here are the faces again. In square A, please write the number of the face that corresponds to the feeling you get when looking at your drawing (SUDS)."*

Note: The clients may write spontaneously what they are feeling: "I am afraid," "I am in danger," and "I can die" = Negative Cognition. It is not necessary to ask the children for it. Just accept what they do in their drawings. The emotional impact doesn't always appear in the first drawing; sometimes it will appear in the second or third one.

Phase 4: Desensitization

Once all of the children have done this, say the following:

Say, *"Please put your crayons aside and do the Butterfly Hug while you are looking at your drawing."*

This lasts for approximately 60 seconds. Some children may need more time (2–3 minutes approximately, or more). Do not interrupt their reprocessing.

Next, the therapist says, *"Now, observe how you feel and draw whatever you want in square B related to the event."*

When they finish drawing in B, the children are shown the faces again.

Say, *"Please look at the faces again and write down the number of the face that corresponds to how you feel when you look at your drawing in square B."*

After writing down the number, say the following:

Say, *"Please put your crayons down and look at your drawing. While you are looking at your drawing, please do the Butterfly Hug."*

This lasts for about 60 seconds.

Next, the therapist says, *"Now, observe how you feel and draw whatever you want in square C related to the event."*

When they finish drawing C, the children are shown the faces again.

Say, *"Please look at the faces again and write down the number of the face that corresponds to how you feel when you look at your drawing in square C."*

After writing down the number, say the following:

Say, *"Please put your crayons down and look at your drawing. While you are looking at your drawing, please do the Butterfly Hug."*

Next, the therapist says, *"Now, observe how you feel and draw whatever you want in square D related to the event."*

When they finish drawing in D, the children are shown the faces again.

Say, *"Please look at the faces again and write down the number of the face that corresponds to how you feel when you look at your drawing in square D."*

After writing down the number, say the following:

Say, *"Please put your crayons down and look at your drawing. While you are looking at your drawing, please do the Butterfly Hug."*

Next, the therapist says, *"Look carefully at the drawing that disturbs you the most. On the back of your paper, where you wrote your name and age, write the number that goes with the face (SUDs) that best describes how you feel about your drawing NOW. Write that number on the upper right hand corner of the paper."*

Phase 5: Future Vision (Instead of Installation)

Phase 5 (Installation) of the standard EMDR Protocol cannot be conducted in large groups for the following reasons: each participant may have a different Subjective Units of Disturbance

(SUD) level because some children can't go any further; are blocking beliefs; have previous problems and trauma; or have different timing for processing (for some it is not enough time to follow the four designs format) and reaching an ecological level of disturbance.

We can do the Installation phase during the individual follow-up intervention (see Phase 8). At this stage of the protocol, we work on a Future Vision to identify adaptive or non-adaptive drawings and cognitions that are helpful in the evaluation of the child at the end of the protocol. An example of a non-adaptive Future Vision: An 8-year-old boy had reported a SUD of 0 when he returned to the target and drew himself in the sky with his dad, God, and angels and he wrote: "I want to die soon to be in the sky with my dad." His mom had told the 8-year-old boy that his dad (who had died in a flood) was very happy in the sky with God and the angels.

Say, *"Now draw how you see yourself in the future."*
Then say, *"Write a word, phrase, or a sentence that explains what you drew."*
Then say, *"Look at your drawing and what you wrote about it and do the Butterfly Hug."*

We believe that if children have an adaptive cognition, the Butterfly Hug will help in their installation and if children do not have an adaptive cognition, the Butterfly Hug will help in the processing to an adaptive state. The EPT monitors this and then gathers all the drawings.

Phase 6: Body Scan

The team leader teaches the children the Body Scan Technique. The therapist says something like the following:

Say, *"Remember the event ... now close your eyes and scan your body from your head to your feet. If you feel any disturbing or pleasant body sensations do the Butterfly Hug and report it to the person who is helping you* (EPT)."

EPT members must identify the children with disturbing body sensations and use that information during Phase 8.

At the end of this exercise the leader says, *"Now move your body like this* (the therapist moves all her body like a dog shaking water off after a bath, making the children laugh)."

This is a fun, play exercise to end on a positive, playful note.

Phase 7: Closure

The therapist then says, *"Go to your Safe Place using the Butterfly Hug."*

Do this for about 60 seconds.

Then say, *"Breathe deeply three times and open your eyes."*

Phase 8: Reevaluation and Follow Up

At the end of the group intervention, the EPT identifies children needing further assistance. These children will need to be thoroughly evaluated to identify the nature and extent of their symptoms, and any co-or preexisting mental health problems. Such a determination is made by taking into consideration reports made by the child's teacher and relatives, the CRTES results, the entire sequence of pictures and SUD Scale ratings, Body Scan, the Future Vision drawing and cognition, and the EPT report.

The team can treat those who require individual follow-up attention, using the EMDR-IGTP in smaller groups than they were in or on an individual basis, keeping in mind the Targeting Sequence Plan and the Three-Pronged Protocol.

SUMMARY SHEET FOR EACH PARTICIPANT:
The EMDR Integrative Group Treatment Protocol (IGTP) for Children

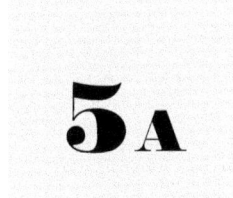

Lucina Artigas, Ignacio Jarero, Nicté Alcalá, and Teresa López Cano
SUMMARY SHEET BY MARILYN LUBER

Name: _____ Diagnosis: _____
Medications: _____
Test Results: _____

The EMDR Integrative Group Treatment Protocol for Children

Phase 1: Client History

Event Date: _____
Event Narrative: _____
_____
_____
_____
_____

☑ Check when task is completed or response has changed or to indicate symptoms.

Phase 2: Preparation—First Part

Introduce Affect (With Dolphin/Another Animal). Animal Makes Face, Then Participant.

☐ Happy ☐ Sad ☐ Scary ☐ Surprised ☐ Angry

Self-Soothing Techniques and the Butterfly Hug—Introduce

Abdominal Breathing: ☐ Completed
Butterfly Hug: ☐ Completed
Safe/Calm Place: ☐ Completed

Assessment of Instrument Administration: ☐ Completed

Phase 2: Preparation—Second Part

Introduce SUD Scale: ☐ Completed

Note: No VoC because there is no Installation Phase

☐ Hand out paper and crayons:
☐ Write name and age on top left:
☐ Divide paper into four parts:

Phase 3: Assessment

☐ Worst part (draw Square A):
☐ SUDs: _____/10
☐ NC (optional):

Phase 4: Desensitization

☐ BH + Look at Drawing A:

☐ Drawing B in Square B:
☐ SUDs in Square B: _____/10
☐ BH + Look at Drawing B:

☐ Drawing C in Square C:
☐ SUDs in Square C: _____/10
☐ BH + Look at Drawing C:

☐ Drawing D in Square D:v
☐ SUDs in Square D: _____/10
☐ BH + Look at Drawing D:

☐ Look at all drawings. Pick the most disturbing. SUDs: _____/10 (upper right-hand corner of name page).

SUDs ratings decrease? ☐ Yes ☐ No

Phase 5: Future Vision (No Installation)

Drawing of self in future: ☐ Completed

Is this drawing adaptive? ☐ Yes ☐ No

Word/phrase/sentence about what is drawn: _____

Is this word/phrase/sentence adaptive? ☐ Yes ☐ No

☐ Look at Future Vision Drawing + BH:
☐ EPT collects drawings.

Phase 6: Body Scan

☐ Body scan + BH: ☐ Completed
☐ Shake body. ☐ Completed

Report a disturbing body sensation? ☐ Yes ☐ No

Phase 7: Closure

☐ Safe place + BH: ☐ Completed
☐ Breathe deeply three times and open your eyes. ☐ Completed

Phase 8: Reevaluation and Follow Up

After taking into consideration the reports made by the child's teacher and relatives, the assessment instruments results, the entire sequence of pictures and SUD Scale ratings, Body Scan, the Future Vision drawing and cognition, and the Emotional Protection Team report, evaluate whether the child/participant needs further help.

Child/participant needs further help? ☐ Yes ☐ No

SUMMARY SHEET FOR CLINICIANS: The EMDR Integrative Group Treatment Protocol (IGTP) for Children

5B

Lucinda Artigas, Ignacio Jarero, Nicté Alcalá, and Teresa López Cano
SUMMARY SHEET BY MARILYN LUBER

Team Leader: _____
EPT: _____
_____
_____
_____

Participants: _____
_____
_____
_____
_____
_____
_____

☑ Check when task is completed or response has changed or to indicate symptoms.

The EMDR Integrative Group Treatment Protocol for Children

Phase 1: Client History

Event Date: _____
Event Narrative: _____
_____
_____
_____
_____

Phase 2: Preparation—First Part

Introduce Affect (with dolphin/another animal)

☐ Happy ☐ Sad ☐ Scary ☐ Surprised ☐ Angry

Self-Soothing Techniques and the Butterfly Hug—Introduce

ABDOMINAL BREATHING: ☐ Completed

☐ Eyes closed + Hand on stomach = Imagine balloon inside stomach.
☐ Inhale (balloon grows and moves hand up).
☐ Exhale (balloon deflates and hand goes down). Observe.

BUTTERFLY HUG: ☐ Completed

Say, *"Please watch me and do what I am doing. Cross your arms over your chest, so that the tip of the middle finger from each hand is placed below the clavicle or the collarbone, and the other fingers and hands cover the area that is located under the connection between the collarbone and the shoulder and the collarbone and sternum or breastbone. Hands and fingers must be as vertical as possible so that the fingers point toward the neck and not toward the arms.*
Now interlock your thumbs to form the butterfly's body and the extension of your other fingers outward will form the butterfly's wings.
Your eyes can be closed, or partially closed, looking toward the tip of your nose. Next, you alternate the movement of your hands, like the flapping wings of a butterfly. Let your hands move freely. You can breathe slowly and deeply (abdominal breathing), *while you observe what is going through your mind and body such as thoughts, images, sounds, odors, feelings, and physical sensations without changing, pushing your thoughts away, or judging. You can pretend as though what you are observing is like clouds passing by."*

SAFE/CALM PLACE: ☐ Completed

Discuss Trauma: ☐ Completed

☐ Validate signs and symptoms: ☐ Completed
☐ Invitation to talk about at home: ☐ Completed

Assessment of Instrument Administration: ☐ Completed

Phase 2: Preparation—Second Part

Introduce SUD scale: ☐ Completed

Note: No VoC because there is no Installation Phase

☐ Hand out paper and crayons:
☐ Write name and age on top left:
☐ Divide paper into four parts:

Phase 3: Assessment

☐ Worst part (draw Square A): ☐ Completed
☐ SUDs: _____/10 ☐ Completed
☐ NC (optional): ☐ Completed

Phase 4: Desensitization

- ☐ BH + Look at Drawing A:

- ☐ Drawing B in Square B:
- ☐ SUDs in Square B: _____/10
- ☐ BH + Look at Drawing B:

- ☐ Drawing C in Square C:
- ☐ SUDs in Square C: _____/10
- ☐ BH + Look at Drawing C:

- ☐ Drawing D in Square D:
- ☐ SUDs in Square D: _____/10
- ☐ BH + Look at Drawing D:

- ☐ Look at all drawings. Pick the most disturbing. SUDs: _____/10 (upper right hand corner of name page).

SUDs ratings decrease? ☐ Yes ☐ No

Phase 5: Future Vision (No Installation) ☐ Completed

- ☐ Drawing of self in future:

Is this drawing adaptive? ☐ Yes ☐ No

Word/phrase/sentence about what drawn: _____

Is this word/phrase/sentence adaptive? ☐ Yes ☐ No

- ☐ Look at Future Vision Drawing + BH:
- ☐ EPT collects drawings.

Phase 6: Body Scan ☐ Completed

- ☐ Body scan + BH:
- ☐ Shake body.

Reports a disturbing body sensation? ☐ Yes ☐ No

Phase 7: Closure ☐ Completed

- ☐ Safe place + BH
- ☐ Breathe deeply three times and open your eyes.

Phase 8: Reevaluation and Follow Up ☐ Completed

Triage (who needs further assistance?): _____

_____

_____

The EMDR Integrative Group Treatment Protocol (IGTP) for Adults

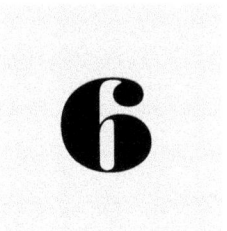

Ignacio Jarero and Lucina Artigas

The EMDR Integrative Group Treatment Protocol (IGTP) Script Notes

The EMDR Integrative Treatment Protocol (IGTP) originally was developed to use with children. The developers have updated the EMDR-IGTP so that it can be used more easily with adults. Changes only occur in Phases 1 and 2 as shown below.

Phase 1: Client History

Working with survivors of man-made and natural catastrophes is a complex issue. First, basic needs such as adequate shelter, food, water, and security for the survivors and their extended families must be addressed. Next, the EMDR-IGTP Team Members must talk and explain to the staff at the shelter, organization, or institution the nature of the work that they are proposing and obtain the authorization to go ahead with the project. After permission is received, it is important for the EMDR-IGTP Team to convene an informal meeting or use another time that has already been designated (i.e., Sunday mass or other scheduled meetings), to explain trauma from an adaptive information processing perspective in as simple language as possible to all the people gathered in the shelter, often 100–300. During this big meeting, the EMDR-IGTP Team extends an invitation to the attendees to participate in a small group process that will help them to reprocess or digest the event. After that, they can inform the attendees of the date, time, and location of the small group process.

It is helpful to know how many people to expect so that appropriate facilities and scheduling can be arranged. If there are not enough team members or facilities for all the people who want to receive support, if possible, schedule several EMDR-IGTP sessions during the following day/s, giving time for the team staff to rest between groups. For a group of 20 to 30 adults, the intervention will take approximately two hours. Also, it is important to take into consideration time and facilities for the one to one work team members may do after the EMDR-IGTP with the participants who need further help.

Say, *"We will have our first group work on ____ (state the date) at ____ (state time) in the ___ (state location). Please come up to any of our team members _____ (point to where the team members are standing) and give them your name and contact information."*

Note: It is essential that team members are aware of the needs of the participants concerning their extended family (e.g., Are the family members safe, are they missing, or did they die?), community (e.g., Did the participants' community organizations such as their church, neighborhood, community associations, schools, or universities survive the catastrophe?), and culture (e.g., Do they need to pray before and after the group or individual psycho-emotional work? Is it culturally accepted to express emotions in public and/or physical demonstrations of compassion/affection?). The team members ask all these types of questions to the shelter staff, such as the General Director, Clinical Director, Physicians, etc., prior to the EMDR-IGTP event.

Phase 2: Preparation—First Part

The professionals who work with survivors of a traumatic event, especially in the immediate aftermath of trauma, should listen actively and supportively, but not probe for details and emotional responses or push for more information than survivors are comfortable providing. Professionals must tread lightly in the wake of disaster so as not to disrupt natural social networks of healing and support. During this protocol, the rest of the team forms an Emotional Protection Team (EPT) around the adults in order to be aware of their emotional reactions and help them when necessary. We recommend a ratio of one team member for every eight to ten adults.

It is important to keep in mind all of the cautions and suggestions in the EMDR IGTP for Children.

If you have a small group of adults (up to 10), prepare the work area by placing enough chairs in a circle for both the survivors and the Emotional Protection Team (EPT). If you have a larger number, participants do not need to be seated in a circle; they can be seated like in a classroom, if this is more comfortable. Welcome the participants and establish rapport with them as they enter the room. Also, it is important to have enough tissues.

The Team Leader introduces him/herself and the members of the EPT:

> Say, *"Hi, my name is* ____ (state name). *I want to introduce you to our Emotional Protection Team. This is* ____ (state name) *and this is* ____ (state name and introduce as many members as there are in the EPT). *We are here to help you with the emotional aspects of* _____ (state the name of the incident). *Thank you for giving us this opportunity to serve you."*

Ask that electronic devices be silenced.

> Say, *"We would appreciate if you would take this opportunity to turn off any electronic devices that you are carrying or put them on vibrate so that we can support the safety in our group today. (Pause) Thank you."*

As in any group, there are basic rules to follow:

> Say, *"In our group today we would like to set up some ways to help our group process today support your healing. With this in mind, we would like you all to agree to not talk about the experience that the other participants speak about to people outside this room.*
> *We ask that you do not take notes, record, or film the group. This is for your benefit only.*
> *We ask that you use this time for your own healing rather than a time to express reproach or assign guilt to other people, as this is not an investigation or a time to criticize yours or anyone's performance.*
> *This is not psychotherapy or a substitute for treatment. This type of work will be available if you or the EPT thinks it would be helpful. Your spoken participation is up to you.*
> *There will be a break at the end of the group process. However, if you need to use the restroom, please do so and return as soon as you can."*

When there is a group of up to 20 participants, ask them to introduce themselves individually:

> Say, *"We would like to invite each one of you to introduce yourselves briefly. Please tell us your name, where you are from, and what happened. Let's start here* ___ (point to participant or say name if it is known) *and then continue around the circle to the right."*

When it is a group of 20 or above, asking each person will take too long, resulting in participants becoming bored and leaving, or the next group will have to leave. It is helpful to wait for spontaneous responses; not all participants need to speak.

> If you are working with a big group, say, *"We would like to invite you to introduce yourselves. Please tell us your name, where you are from, and what happened?"*

If culturally appropriate, ask for a volunteer to lead the group in prayer:

> Say, *"I would like to ask who would like to volunteer to lead us in prayer?" (Pause). "Thank you ____ (state name of volunteer), please go ahead."*

Introduce the Adaptive Information Processing System (AIP) and ask for the types of symptoms that the participants have. This part is for screening or triage that may later lead to one on one intervention, as needed. It is important not to force anyone to talk.

> Say, *"Thank you, ____ (state name). Now, I would like to explain to you the basis upon which we have built our experience for today, We call it the Adaptive Information Processing (AIP) system and it helps us to digest what has happened to us in the same way we can digest a light meal with no problem, but we often have difficulty when we eat heavy food that is hard to digest. Frequently, we can have a number of symptoms when that happens. What do you notice when you have eaten a meal that is too heavy or too much for you?"* (Wait for responses).

> Say, *"That is right. In the same manner, heavy information such as ___ (state the nature of the critical incident) is difficult for the brain to digest and causes symptoms. What symptoms have you noticed since the day of the event until now?"*

Note: Pay attention to the symptoms of deterioration or dysfunction (such as participants who are unable to tend to their basic responsibilities and/or perform daily activities) because they will play an important role in triaging/selecting who will be invited to receive personal attention at the conclusion of the EMDR-IGTP.

When everyone has finished speaking, the leader, or a co-leader selected beforehand, normalizes symptoms by saying the following:

> Say, *"The symptoms that you all mentioned are normal. They are the kinds of reactions normal people have after an abnormal experience such as _____ (state the critical incident)."*

Note: If 30 days have already gone by since the critical incident occurred, we do not say that the symptoms are normal (since they are not), but rather we say:

> Say, *"All of the symptoms that you have mentioned are ways your brain's processing system is trying to assimilate this experience."*

Mention the availability of staff for further help.

> Say, *"I also want to remind you that all of us will be available to you after our experience today and at other times. We would be honored to continue to help you—and others you know—in any way that we can."*

Teach Self-Soothing Exercises

> Say, *"Our next exercise is one that will help all of us learn to soothe ourselves. During the exercise the Emotional Protection Team will take care of*

everything, so you are welcome to relax and close your eyes if you would like to do so."

Let one of the EPT lead the following exercises:

ABDOMINAL BREATHING

Say, *"Close your eyes put one hand on your stomach and imagine that you have a balloon inside your stomach. Now, inhale and see how the balloon grows and moves your hand up. Now you can exhale and see how the balloon deflates, and, your hand goes down. Put all your attention in that. If anything distracts you gently return to the exercise."*

Do this exercise for 5 minutes.

CONCENTRATION EXERCISE (5 MINUTES)

Say, *"I would like you to take a little time to think about your breathing. Notice when you are inhaling and say to yourself, 'I am inhaling,' and then notice when you are exhaling and say to yourself, 'I am exhaling.' Continue to allow your attention to focus on your breath, for a while longer, gently bringing yourself back—if you are distracted—to the inhaling and exhaling of your breath."*

Do this exercise for 5 minutes.

PLEASANT MEMORY

Say, *"Remember a time when you were calm or happy. (Pause). Now, put your hand on your chest and let those good feelings and positive physical sensations expand throughout your body. Good. Continue to allow your attention to focus on these good feelings and sensations for a while longer, gently bringing yourself back—if you are distracted—to the happy and calm feelings you are feeling."*

At the end, say, *"As you open your eyes, remember that in the future all you have to do to bring back the memory is to place your hand over the center of your chest."*

Do this exercise for 5 minutes.

THE BUTTERFLY HUG

Say, *"Would you like to learn an exercise that will help you to feel better?"*

Say, *"Please watch me and do what I am doing. Cross your arms over your chest, so that the tip of the middle finger from each hand is placed below the clavicle or the collarbone, and the other fingers and hands cover the area that is located under the connection between the collarbone and the shoulder and the collarbone and sternum or breastbone. Hands and fingers must be as vertical as possible so that the fingers point toward the neck and not toward the arms.*

Now interlock your thumbs to form the butterfly's body and the extension of your other fingers outward will form the butterfly s wings. Your eyes can be closed, or partially closed, looking toward the tip of your nose. Next, you alternate the movement of your hands, like the flapping wings of a butterfly. Let your hands move freely. You can breathe slowly and deeply (abdominal breathing), *while you observe what is going through your mind and body such as thoughts, images, sounds, odors, feelings, and physical sensations without changing, pushing your thoughts away, or judging. You can pretend as though what you are observing is like clouds passing by."*

It is important to observe the participants to make sure that they are able to follow along with you. If not, members of the EPT can be alert and quietly go up to a participant to help as needed and then return to teaching the Butterfly Hug.

At the end, say: *"In the future, if you experience an ongoing, highly distressing stressor and your self-soothing techniques fail to help you to calm down quickly, do the Butterfly Hug to help process the current situation."*

The Team Leader asks participants how they are feeling:

Say, *"We have just practiced different ways to soothe ourselves and I am wondering how you are feeling now?"*

The Team Leader explains coping strategies:

Say, *"After a traumatic event such as the _____* (state event) *that all of you have been through, it is helpful to make sure that you do some things that may seem pretty basic but are really important such as drinking a lot of water even when you are not thirsty, eating healthy foods, making sure to exercise* (but not overdoing it), *and taking short breaks during the day in order to practice your self-soothing techniques such as abdominal breathing, the concentration exercise, or the pleasant memory technique."*

Say, *"Do any of you have any questions that you would like to ask me or the members of the Emotional Protection Team?"*

Trauma Work

Say, *"At the beginning of this work, you mentioned the symptoms that you noticed since the day of the event until now. We want to remind you that all of the symptoms you have mentioned are ways your brain's processing system is trying to assimilate this experience. It is also normal to have different feelings than your friends and other people, since each person experiences and feels things differently."*

The facilitator goes on and says, *"When you return home after this exercise, you can talk to the people you trust about your thoughts and feelings, as much as you want and when you feel most comfortable doing so."*

The aim is to verbalize the traumatic memories and to respond to the acute need that arises in many survivors to share their experience, while at the same time respecting their natural inclination with regard to how much, when, and to whom they talk.

At the end of this first part of the Preparation Phase, the team administers the appropriate measures (e.g., Impact of Event Scale [IES], Impact of Event Scale-Revised [IES-R], or any other valid measure).

Say, *"Here is a scale for you to look at. Please answer the questions on it. If you have any questions, please ask one of the Emotional Protection Team Members to help you out."*

Note: Standardized psychological assessment is used cautiously. It is helpful for team members to be concerned about the rapport with the participants. They need to demonstrate by their behavior that they are truly interested in them as human beings and not as objects of scientific curiosity. This custom weakens the scientific value of data gathered, while it respects the wishes of our Latin American clients not to be stigmatized by formal testing procedures. In our experience, clients also tend to reject assistance from those they judge to be opportunists, in this case anyone who seems interested in the victim as an object of study.

Phase 2: Preparation—Second Part

It is important to use language that the participants can understand. In countries where cultural development is not as advanced, it may be helpful to utilize the language that is used with children, adolescents, etc. in order to assist participants with the task.

Show the participants the faces that measure SUDs from 0 to 10, with 0 being no disturbance, and 10 being maximum disturbance. If you do not have the original faces you can draw them on the blackboard.

> Say, *"Here are faces that measure our feelings on a 0 to 10 scale, where 0 does not bother you at all and 10 bothers you the most possible."*

Note: Clinicians are welcome to use the best words and pictures possible for their population.

Familiarize the participants with the scale.

> Say, *"How do you feel when you do a good job? Please point to the face that describes how you feel."*
>
> Now say, *"How do you feel when you are sick? Please point to the face that tells us how you feel."*

We have observed that participants who are not yet familiar with the numbers will sometimes say a number and point to a face that does not correspond. Thus, it is better to pick the face they point to over the number they say (one of the members of the EPT can write the correct number). The members of the EPT hand out white pieces of paper and crayons to each of the participants (have extra crayons in case the participants ask for more).

> Say, *"Please write your name and age on the top left side of the paper* (show how to do it).*"*

EPT members can aid those who cannot do it.

> Say, *"Now, please divide the other side of the paper in four equal parts like this. Draw a cross at the center like this and write a small letter at the top left corner of each section like this."*

The therapist shows them how to do it on the blackboard and the EPT helps.

Note: Often, we had to divide the sheet of paper in four, given the scarcity of the materials in the shelters, but it is acceptable to use four sheets of paper, making sure that each has the name and the age of the participant and the corresponding letter, so that the sequence can be identified.

Phase 3: Assessment

The therapist says, *"Whoever remembers what happened during the event _____ (mention the event—hurricane, flooding, explosion, etc.), please raise your hands."*
The participants raise their hands.

> Say, *"Now, close your eyes and observe what makes you the most frightened, sad, or angry about that event _____ (mention the event) NOW."*

The therapist continues, *"Take whatever emerges from your head to your neck, to your arms, to your hands and fingers, to the crayon, and now open your eyes and draw it in square A."*

When all the participants are finished, show them the faces again.

Say, *"Here are the faces again. In square A, please write the number of the face that corresponds to the feeling you get when looking at your drawing (SUDS)."*

Note: The participants may write spontaneously what they are feeling: "I am afraid," "I am in danger," "I can die" = Negative Cognition. It is not necessary to ask the participants for it. Just accept what they do in their drawing. The emotional impact doesn't always appear in the first drawing; sometimes it will appear in the second or third one.

Phase 4: Desensitization

Once all of the participants have done this, say the following:

Say, *"Please put your crayons aside and do the Butterfly Hug while you are looking at your drawing."*

This lasts for approximately 60 seconds.

Next, the therapist says, *"Now, observe how you feel and draw whatever you want in square B related to the event."*

When they finish drawing in B, the participants are shown the faces again.

Say, *"Please look at the faces again and write down the number of the face that corresponds to how you feel when you look at your drawing in square B."*

After writing down the number, say the following:

Say, *"Please put your crayons down and look at your drawing. While you are looking at your drawing, please do the Butterfly Hug."*

This lasts for about 60 seconds.

Next, the therapist says, *"Now, observe how you feel and draw whatever you want in square C related to the event."*

When they finish drawing C, the participants are shown the faces again.

Say, *"Please look at the faces again and write down the number of the face that corresponds to how you feel when you look at your drawing in square C."*

After writing down the number, say the following:

Say, *"Please put your crayons down and look at your drawing. While you are looking at your drawing, please do the Butterfly Hug."*

Next, the therapist says, *"Now, observe how you feel and draw whatever you want in square D related to the event."*

When they finish drawing in D, the participants are shown the faces again.

Say, *"Please look at the faces again and write down the number of the face that corresponds to how you feel when you look at your drawing in square D."*

After writing down the number, say the following:

Say, *"Please put your crayons down and look at your drawing. While you are looking at your drawing, please do the Butterfly Hug."*

Next, the therapist says, *"Look carefully at the drawing that disturbs you the most. On the back of your paper, where you wrote your name and age, write the number that goes with the face (SUDs) that best describes how you feel about your drawing NOW. Write that number on the upper right hand corner of the paper."*

Phase 5: Future Vision (Instead of Installation)

Phase 5 (Installation) of the Standard EMDR Protocol cannot be conducted in large groups for the following reasons: each participant may have a different SUD level because some participants can't go any further; blocking beliefs; previous problems and trauma; or have different timing for processing (for some it is not enough time to follow the four designs format) and reach an ecological level of disturbance.

We can do the Installation Phase during the individual follow-up intervention (see Phase 8). At this stage of the protocol, we work on a Future Vision to identify adaptive or non-adaptive drawings and cognitions that are helpful in the evaluation of the participant at the end of the protocol. An example of a non-adaptive Future Vision in an adult is if he does not see a future for himself, as when a 28-year-old man drew a black circle and wrote "I have nothing to do in the future."

> Say, *"Now draw how you see yourself in the future."*
> Then say, *"Write a word, phrase, or a sentence that explains what you drew."*
> Then say, *"Look at your drawing and what you wrote about it and do the Butterfly Hug."*

We believe that if participants have an adaptive cognition, the Butterfly Hug will help in their installation and if the participant does not have an adaptive cognition, the Butterfly Hug will help in the processing to an adaptive state. The EPT monitors this and then gathers all the drawings.

Phase 6: Body Scan

The team leader teaches the participants the Body Scan Technique. The therapist says something like the following:

> Say, *"Remember the event... Now, close your eyes and scan your body from your head to your feet. If you feel any disturbing or pleasant body sensations do the Butterfly Hug and report it to the person who is helping you (EPT)."*

EPT members identify participants with disturbing body sensations and use that information during Phase 8.

At the end of this exercise the leader says, *"Now move your body like this* (the therapist moves all of his/her body like a dog shaking water off after a bath, making the participants laugh)."

This is a fun, play exercise to end on a positive, playful note.

Phase 7: Closure

> The therapist then says, *"Go to your Safe Place using the Butterfly Hug."*
> Do this for about 60 seconds.
> Then say, *"Breathe deeply three times and open your eyes."*

Phase 8: Reevaluation and Follow Up

At the end of the group intervention, the EPT identifies participants needing further assistance. These participants will need to be thoroughly evaluated to identify the nature and extent of their symptoms, and any co-or preexisting mental health problems. Staff can make this determination by taking into consideration reports made by the participants' relatives and/or friends, whatever valid measure is used (i.e., IES, IES-R), the entire sequence of pictures, the SUD Scale ratings, Body Scan, the Future Vision drawing and cognition, and the Emotional Protection Team Report.

The team can treat those who require individual follow-up attention using the EMDR-IGTP in smaller groups than they were in or on an individual basis, keeping in mind the Targeting Sequence Plan and the Three-Pronged Protocol.

SUMMARY SHEET FOR EACH PARTICIPANT:
The EMDR Integrative Group Treatment Protocol (IGTP) for Adults

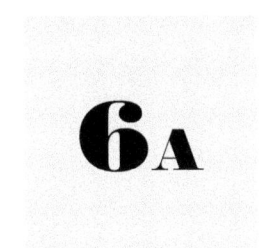

Ignacio Jarero and Lucina Artigas
SUMMARY SHEET BY MARILYN LUBER

Name: _____ Diagnosis: _____
Medications: _____
Test Results: _____

☑ Check when task is completed or response has changed or to indicate symptoms.

The EMDR Integrative Group Treatment Protocol for Adults

Phase 1: Client History

Event Date: _____
Event Narrative: _____
_____
_____
_____
_____

Phase 2: Preparation—First Part

Self-Soothing Techniques and the Butterfly Hug—Introduction

Abdominal Breathing:	☐ Completed
Concentration Exercise	☐ Completed
Pleasant Memory	☐ Completed
Butterfly Hug:	☐ Completed
Safe/Calm Place:	☐ Completed

Assessment Instrument Administration ☐ Completed

Phase 2: Preparation—Second Part

Introduce SUD Scale: ☐ Completed

Note: No VoC because there is no Installation Phase

☐ Hand out paper and crayons:	☐ Completed
☐ Write name and age on top left:	☐ Completed
☐ Divide paper in four parts:	☐ Completed

Phase 3: Assessment

- ☐ Worst Part (Draw Square A):
- ☐ SUDs: ____/10
- ☐ NC (optional):

Phase 4: Desensitization

- ☐ BH + Look at Drawing A:

- ☐ Drawing B in Square B:
- ☐ SUDs in Square B: ____/10
- ☐ BH + Look at Drawing B:

- ☐ Drawing C in Square C:
- ☐ SUDs in Square C: ____/10
- ☐ BH + Look at Drawing C

- ☐ Drawing D in Square D:
- ☐ SUDs in Square D: ____/10
- ☐ BH + Look at Drawing D
- ☐ Look at all drawings. Pick most disturbing. SUDs: ____/10 (upper right hand corner of name page).

SUDs ratings decrease? ☐ Yes ☐ No

Phase 5: Future Vision (No Installation)

Drawing of self in future: ☐ Completed

Is this drawing adaptive? ☐ Yes ☐ No

Word/phrase/sentence about what drawn: _____

Is this word/phrase/sentence adaptive? ☐ Yes ☐ No

- ☐ Look at Future Drawing + BH:
- ☐ EPT collects drawings.

Phase 6: Body Scan

- ☐ Body Scan + BH:
- ☐ Shake body.

Report a disturbing body sensation? ☐ Yes ☐ No

Phase 7: Closure

- ☐ Safe Place + BH:
- ☐ Breathe deeply three times and open your eyes.

Phase 8: Reevaluation and Follow Up

At the end of the group intervention, the EPT identifies participants needing further assistance. These participants will need to be thoroughly evaluated to identify the nature and extent of their symptoms and any co- or preexisting mental health problems. Staff can make this determination by taking into consideration reports made by the participants' relatives and/or friends, whatever valid measure is used (i.e., IES, IES-R), the entire sequence of pictures, the SUD Scale ratings, Body Scan, the Future Vision drawing and cognition, and the Emotional Protection Team Report.

Participant needs further help? ☐ Yes ☐ No

SUMMARY SHEET FOR CLINICIANS: The EMDR Integrative Group Treatment Protocol (IGTP) for Adults

6B

Ignacio Jarero and Lucina Artigas
SUMMARY SHEET BY MARILYN LUBER

Name: _____ Diagnosis: _____

Medications: _____

Test Results: _____

☑ Check when task is completed or response has changed or to indicate symptoms.

The EMDR Integrative Group Treatment Protocol for Adults

Phase 1: Client History

Event Date: _____

Event Narrative: _____

_____

_____

_____

_____

Phase 2: Preparation—First Part

☐ Introduce confidentiality:
☐ Introduction of each member:
☐ Discuss AIP:

Introduce Self-Soothing Techniques and the Butterfly Hug.

ABDOMINAL BREATHING ☐ Completed

☐ Eyes Closed + Hand on Stomach = Imagine Balloon inside Stomach.
☐ Inhale (balloon grows and moves hand up).
☐ Exhale (balloon deflates and hand goes down). Observe

CONCENTRATION EXERCISE   ☐ Completed

> Say, *"I would like you to take a little time to think about your breathing. Notice when you are inhaling and say to yourself, 'I am inhaling,' and then notice when you are exhaling and say to yourself, 'I am exhaling.' Continue to allow your attention to focus on your breath, for a while longer, gently bringing yourself back—if you are distracted—to the inhaling and exhaling of your breath."*

> Do this exercise for 5 minutes.

PLEASANT MEMORY   ☐ Completed

> Say, *"Remember a time when you were calm or happy. (Pause). Now, put your hand on your chest and let those good feelings and positive physical sensations expand throughout your body. Good. Continue to allow your attention to focus on these good feelings and sensations for a while longer, gently bringing yourself back—if you are distracted—to the happy and calm feelings you are feeling."*
> At the end, say, *"As you open your eyes, remember that in the future all you have to do to bring back the memory is to place your hand over the center of your chest."* Do this exercise for 5 minutes.

THE BUTTERFLY HUG   ☐ Completed

> Say, *"Please watch me and do what I am doing. Cross your arms over your chest, so that the tip of the middle finger from each hand is placed below the clavicle or the collarbone and the other fingers and hands cover the area that is located under the connection between the collarbone and the shoulder and the collarbone and sternum or breastbone. Hands and fingers must be as vertical as possible so that the fingers point toward the neck and not toward the arms. Now interlock your thumbs to form the butterfly's body and the extension of your other fingers outward will form the butterfly's wings. Your eyes can be closed, or partially closed, looking toward the tip of your nose. Next, you alternate the movement of your hands, like the flapping wings of a butterfly. Let your hands move freely. You can breathe slowly and deeply [abdominal breathing], while you observe what is going through your mind and body such as thoughts, images, sounds, odors, feelings, and physical sensations without changing, pushing your thoughts away, or judging. You can pretend as though what you are observing is like clouds passing by."*

SAFE/CALM PLACE   ☐ Completed

Discuss Trauma   ☐ Completed

    ☐ Validate Signs and Symptoms:
    ☐ Invitation to talk about at home:

Assessment Instrument Administration   ☐ Completed

Phase 2: Preparation—Second Part

Introduce SUD Scale:

Note: No VoC because there is no Installation Phase

    ☐ Hand out paper and crayons:
    ☐ Write name and age on top left:
    ☐ Divide paper in four parts: ☐ Completed

Phase 3: Assessment ☐ Completed

- ☐ Worst Part (Draw Square A):
- ☐ SUDs: ___/10
- ☐ NC (optional):

Phase 4: Desensitization ☐ Completed

- ☐ BH + Look at Drawing A:

- ☐ Drawing B in Square B:
- ☐ SUDs in Square B:___/10
- ☐ BH + Look at Drawing B:

- ☐ Drawing C in Square C:
- ☐ SUDs in Square C: ___/10
- ☐ BH + Look at Drawing C

- ☐ Drawing D in Square D:
- ☐ SUDs in Square D: ___/10
- ☐ BH + Look at Drawing D

Look at all drawings. Pick most disturbing. SUDs:___/10 (upper right hand corner of name page).

SUDs ratings decrease? ☐ Yes ☐ No

Phase 5: Future Vision (No Installation) ☐ Completed

- ☐ Drawing of self in future:

Is this drawing adaptive? ☐ Yes ☐ No

Word/phrase/sentence about what drawn: _____

Is this word/phrase/sentence adaptive? ☐ Yes ☐ No

- ☐ Look at Future Vision Drawing + BH:
- ☐ EPT collects drawings.

Phase 6: Body Scan ☐ Completed

- ☐ Body Scan + BH:
- ☐ Shake body.

Report a disturbing body sensation? ☐ Yes ☐ No

Phase 7: Closure ☐ Completed

- ☐ Safe Place + BH:
- ☐ Breathe deeply three times and open your eyes.

Phase 8: Reevaluation and Follow Up ☐ Completed

At the end of the group intervention, the EPT identifies participants needing further assistance. These participants will need to be thoroughly evaluated to identify the nature and extent of their symptoms, and any co-or preexisting mental health problems. Staff can make this determination by taking into consideration reports made by the participants' relatives and/or friends, whatever valid measure used (i.e., IES, IES-R), the entire sequence of pictures, the SUD Scale ratings, Body Scan, the Future Vision drawing and cognition, and the Emotional Protection Team Report.

Participant needs further help. ☐ Yes ☐ No

Appendix A: Worksheets

Past Memory Worksheet Script (Shapiro, 2001, 2006)

Phase 3: Assessment

Incident

Say, *"The memory that we will start with today is _____ (select the next incident to be targeted)."*

_____
_____
_____

Say, *"What happens when you think of the _____ (state the issue)?"*

_____
_____
_____

Or say, *"When you think of _____ (state the issue), what do you get?"*

_____
_____

Picture

Say, *"What picture represents the entire _____ (state the issue)?"*

_____
_____
_____

If there are many choices or if the client becomes confused, the clinician assists by asking the following:

Say, *"What picture represents the most traumatic part of _____ (state the issue)?"*

_____
_____

Negative Cognition (NC)

Say, *"What words best go with the picture that express your negative belief about yourself now?"*

_____

_____

Positive Cognition (PC)

Say, *"When you bring up that picture or _____ (state the issue), what would you like to believe about yourself now?"*

_____

_____

Validity of Cognition (VoC)

Say, *"When you think of the incident (or picture) how true do those words ____ (clinician repeats the positive cognition) feel to you now on a scale of 1 to 7, where 1 feels completely false and 7 feels completely true?"*

  1   2   3   4   5   6   7
(completely false)   (completely true)

Emotions

Say, *"When you bring up the picture or _____ (state the issue) and those words ____ (clinician states the negative cognition), what emotion do you feel now?"*

_____

Subjective Units of Disturbance (SUD)

Say, *"On a scale of 0 to 10, where 0 is no disturbance or neutral and 10 is the highest disturbance you can imagine, how disturbing does it feel now?"*

  0   1   2   3   4   5   6   7   8   9   10
(no disturbance)   (highest disturbance)

Location of Body Sensation

Say, *"Where do you feel it (the disturbance) in your body?"*

_____

Phase 4: Desensitization

To begin, say the following:

Say, *"Now, remember, it is your own brain that is doing the healing and you are the one in control. I will ask you to mentally focus on the target and to follow my fingers (or any other BLS you are using). Just let whatever happens, happen, and we will talk at the end of the set. Just tell me what comes up, and don't discard anything as unimportant. Any new information that comes to mind is connected in some way. If you want to stop, just raise your hand."*

Then say, *"Bring up the picture and the words _____ (clinician repeats the NC) and notice where you feel it in your body. Now follow my fingers with your eyes (or other BLS)."*

Phase 5: Installation

Say, *"How does _____ (repeat the PC) sound?"*

_____
_____
_____

Say, *"Do the words _____ (repeat the PC) still fit, or is there another positive statement that feels better?"*

_____
_____
_____

If the client accepts the original positive cognition, the clinician should ask for a VoC rating to see if it has improved:

Say, *"As you think of the incident, how do the words feel, from 1 (completely false) to 7 (completely true)?"*

1   2   3   4   5   6   7
(completely false)   (completely true)

Say, *"Think of the event and hold it together with the words _____ (repeat the PC)."*

Do a long set of bilateral stimulation (BLS) to see if there is more processing to be done.

Phase 6: Body Scan

Say, *"Close your eyes and keep in mind the original memory and the positive cognition. Then bring your attention to the different parts of your body, starting with your head and working downward. Any place you find any tension, tightness, or unusual sensation, tell me."*

_____
_____

Phase 7: Closure

Say, *"Things may come up or they may not. If they do, great. Write it down and it can be a target for next time. You can use a log to write down what triggers images, thoughts or cognitions, emotions, and sensations; you can rate them on our 0 to 10 scale where 0 is no disturbance or neutral and 10 is the worst disturbance. Please write down the positive experiences, too."*

"If you get any new memories, dreams, or situations that disturb you, just take a good snapshot. It isn't necessary to give a lot of detail. Just put down enough to remind you so we can target it next time. The same thing goes for any positive dreams or situations. If negative feelings do come up, try not to make them significant. Remember, it's still just the old stuff. Just write it down for next time. Then use the tape or the Safe Place exercise to let as much of the disturbance go as possible. Even if nothing comes up, make sure to use the tape every day and give me a call if you need to."

Phase 8: Reevaluation

There are four ways to reevaluate our work with clients.

1. Reevaluate Since the Last Session

Reevaluate what has come up in the client's life since the last session.

Say, *"Okay. Let's look at your log. I am interested in what has happened since the last session. What have you noticed since our last session?"*

_____
_____
_____

Say, *"What has changed?"*

_____
_____
_____

If the client has nothing to say or does not say much, say the following:

Say, *"Have you had any dreams or nightmares?"*

_____
_____

Say, *"What about _____ (state symptoms you and client have been working on) we have been working on, have you noticed any changes in them? Have they increased or decreased?"*

_____
_____

Say, *"Have you noticed any other changes, new responses, or insights in your images, thoughts, emotions, sensations, and behaviors?"*

_____
_____

Say, *"Have you found new resources?"*

_____
_____
_____

Say, *"Have any situations, events, or other stimuli triggered you?"*

_____
_____
_____

Use the material from your reevaluation to feed back into your case conceptualization and help decide what to do next concerning the larger treatment plan.

2. Reevaluate The Previous Target

Reevaluate the target worked on in the previous session. Has the individual target been resolved? Whether the previous processing session was complete or incomplete, use the following instructions to access the memory and determine the need for further processing.

Say, *"Bring up the memory or trigger of _____ (state the memory or trigger) that we worked on last session. What image comes up?"*

_____
_____
_____

Say, *"What thoughts about it come up?"*

_____
_____

Say, *"What thoughts about yourself?"*

_____
_____

Say, *"What emotions do you notice?"*

_____
_____

Say, *"What sensations do you notice?"*

_____
_____

Say, *"On a scale of 0 to 10, where 0 is no disturbance or neutral and 10 is the highest disturbance you can imagine, how disturbing does it feel now?"*

0   1   2   3   4   5   6   7   8   9   10
(no disturbance)   (highest disturbance)

Evaluate the material to see if there are any indications of dysfunction. Has the primary issue been resolved? Is there ecological validity to the client's resolution of the issue? Is there associated material that has been activated that must be addressed?

If you are observing any resistance to resolving the issue, say the following:

Say, *"What would happen if you are successful?"*

_____
_____

If there are no indications of dysfunction, and SUD is 0, do a set of BLS to be sure that the processing is complete.

Say, *"Go with that."*

Say, *"What do you get now?"*

_____
_____

Check the positive cognition.

Say, "*When you think of the incident* (or picture) *how true do those words* _____ (clinician repeats the positive cognition) *feel to you now on a scale of 1 to 7, where 1 feels completely false and 7 feels completely true?*"

1   2   3   4   5   6   7
(completely false)   (completely true)

If the VoC is 7, do a set of BLS to be sure that the processing is complete.

Say, *"Go with that."*

Say, *"What do you get now?"*

_____

_____

If there are any signs of dysfunction such as a new negative perspective(s) or new facets of the event or the SUD is higher than 0, say the following:

Say, *"Okay, now please pay attention to the image, thoughts, and sensations associated with* _____ (state the memory or trigger) *and just go with that."*

_____

_____

Continue with the Standard EMDR Protocol until processing is complete.

If the VoC is less than 7, say the following:

Say, "*What is keeping it from being a 7?*"

_____

_____

Note the associated feelings and sensations, and resume processing.

Say, *"Go with that."*

Continue with the Standard EMDR Protocol through the Body Scan until processing is complete.

If a completely new incident or target emerges, say the following:

Say, *"Are there any feeder memories contributing to this problem?"*

_____

_____

Do the Assessment Phase on the appropriate target and fully process it. It is not unusual for another aspect of the memory to emerge that needs to be processed.

If the client claims that nothing or no disturbance is coming up (or he can't remember what was worked on in the previous session), and the therapist thinks that the work is probably still incomplete and that the client is simply not able to access the memory, say the following:

Say, *"When you think of* _____ (state the incident that was worked on) *and the image* _____ (state the image) *and* _____ (state the NC), *what body sensations do you feel now?"*

_____

_____

Say, *"Go with that"*.

_____

_____

Continue processing with the Standard EMDR Protocol.

If the client wants to work on a *charged* trigger that came up since the last session instead of the target from the previous session, say the following:

Say, *"Yes, this IS important information. Tell me about what came up for you."*

_____

_____

Then assess the magnitude of the trigger. If it is indeed a severe critical incident, then proceed accordingly, using the Assessment Phase to target the new material and return to the original target when possible.

If it is not, then say the following:

Say, *"Yes this is important, however, it is important that we finish our work on _____ (state what you are working on) before moving to another target. It is like what happens when you have too many files open on your computer and it slows down, or finishing the course of antibiotics even if you feel okay (or any other appropriate metaphor for your client)."*

Fully reprocess each target through the Body Scan and Reevaluation before moving on to the next in order to ensure optimal results.

3. Reevaluate at Critical Points

At various critical points in treatment (before moving on to the next symptom, theme, goal, etc.), reevaluate what has been effectively targeted and resolved and what still needs to be addressed.

Say, *"Now that we have finished this work, let's reevaluate our work so far. Remember _____ (state the work you have done). On a scale of 0 to 10, where 0 is no disturbance or neutral and 10 is the highest disturbance you can imagine, how disturbing does it feel now?"*

0	1	2	3	4	5	6	7	8	9	10
(no disturbance)										(highest disturbance)

If the SUD is higher than 0, evaluate what else needs to be done by continuing to work with the disturbance in the framework of the Standard EMDR Protocol.

Also evaluate whether the client has been able to achieve cognitive, behavioral, and emotional goals in his life.

Say, *"Have you accomplished all of the goals that we had contracted to work on such as _____ (read the list of agreed upon goals)?"*

_____

_____

_____

If not, evaluate what still needs to be targeted such as feeder memories.

Say, *"Please scan for an earlier memory that incorporates _____ (state the negative cognition). What do you get?"*

_____

_____

Use the Standard EMDR Protocol to process any feeder memories.
Check if previously identified clusters of memories remain charged.

Say, *"Are there any memories left concerning* _____ *(state the cluster of memories previously worked on)?"*

_____

_____

_____

If so, work on the memory(ies), using the Standard EMDR Protocol. Make sure to incorporate the positive templates for all previously disturbing situations and projected future goals. See the Future Template Worksheet Script.

4. Reevaluate Before Termination

Before termination, reevaluate targets worked on over the course of therapy and goals addressed during treatment.

Say, *"Before we end our treatment, let's reevaluate our work to make sure that all of the targets are resolved and goals are addressed. Are there any PAST targets that remain unresolved for you?"*

_____

_____

_____

Or say, *"These are the past targets with which we worked; do any of them remain unresolved? What about the memories that we listed during our history taking and over the course of treatment?"*

_____

_____

_____

Check with the SUDs for any disturbance.

Say, *"On a scale of 0 to 10, where 0 is no disturbance or neutral and 10 is the highest disturbance you can imagine, how disturbing does it feel now?"*

0   1   2   3   4   5   6   7   8   9   10
(no disturbance)   (highest disturbance)

Check the major negative cognitions to see if there are any unresolved memories still active.

Say, *"These are the main negative cognitions with which we worked. Hold* _____ *(state one of the cognitions worked with) and scan for any unresolved memories. Does anything surface for you?"*

_____

_____

If there is more unresolved material, check with BLS to see if the charge decreases. If not, use the Standard EMDR Protocol.

Say, *"Now scan chronologically from birth until today to see if there are any other unresolved memories. What do you notice?"*

_____

_____

If there is more unresolved material, check with BLS to see if the charge decreases. If not, use the Standard EMDR Protocol.

Progressions can occur during other events or during the processing of a primary target; use your clinical judgment as to whether it is important to return and reevaluate these memories.

Clusters are related memories that were grouped together during treatment planning and can be scanned to identify any memories that were not involved through generalization of treatment effects.

Say, *"Let's check the _____ (state the cluster) we worked on earlier. When you think about it are there any other memories that were not involved that you are aware of now?"*

_____

_____

If there is more unresolved material, check with BLS to see if the charge decreases. If not, use the Standard EMDR Protocol.

Participants are significant individuals in the client's life who should be targeted if memories or issues regarding them remain disturbing.

Say, *"Let's check if there are any remaining concerns or memories concerning ____ (state whoever the client might be concerned about). Is there anything that still is bothering you about _____ (state the person's name)?"*

_____

_____

If there is more unresolved material, check with BLS to see if the charge decreases. If not, use the Standard EMDR Protocol.

Say, *"Are there any PRESENT or RECENT triggers that remain potent?"*

_____

_____

_____

Say, *"Are there any current conditions, situations, or people that make you want to avoid them, act in ways that are not helpful, or cause you emotional distress?"*

_____

_____

If there is more unresolved material, check with BLS to see if the charge decreases. If not, use the Standard EMDR Protocol.

Say, *"Are there any future goals that have not been addressed and realized?"*

_____

_____

Make sure to use the Future Template for each trigger, new goal(s), new skill(s), issues of memory, or incorporating the client's new sense of himself. See Future Template Worksheet Script in this appendix.

Present Trigger Worksheet Script

Target and reprocess present triggers identified during History Taking, reprocessing, and reevaluation. Steps for working with present triggers are the following.

1. Identify the presenting trigger that is still causing disturbance.
2. Target and activate the presenting trigger using the full Assessment procedures (image, negative cognition, positive cognition, VoC, emotions, SUD, sensations).
3. Follow Phases 3 through 8 with each trigger until it is fully reprocessed (SUD = 0, VoC = 7, clear Body Scan) before moving to the next trigger.

   Note: In some situations a blocking belief may be associated with the present trigger requiring a new Targeting Sequence Plan.

4. Once all present triggers have been reprocessed, proceed to installing Future Templates for each present trigger (e.g., imagining encountering the same situation in the future; see Future Template protocols).

Present Stimuli That Trigger the Disturbing Memory or Reaction

List the situations that elicit the symptom(s). Examples of situations, events, or stimuli that trigger clients could be the following: another trauma, the sound of a car backfiring, or being touched in a certain way.

Say, *"What are the situations, events, or stimuli that trigger your trauma _____ (state the trauma). Let's process these situations, events, or stimuli triggers one-by-one."*

Situations, Events, or Stimuli Trigger List

_____
_____
_____
_____
_____

Target or Memory

Say, *"What situation, event, or stimulus that triggers you would you like to use as a target today?"*

_____
_____

Picture

Say, *"What picture represents the _____ (state the situation, event, or stimulus) that triggers you?"*

_____
_____

If there are many choices or if the client becomes confused, the clinician assists by asking the following:

Say, *"What picture represents the most traumatic part of the _____ (state the situation, event, or stimulus) that triggers you?"*

_____

_____

When a picture is unavailable, the clinician merely invites the client to do the following:

Say, *"Think of the _____ (state the situation, event, or stimulus) that triggers you."*

_____

_____

Negative Cognition (NC)

Say, *"What words best go with the picture that express your negative belief about yourself now?"*

_____

Positive Cognition (PC)

Say, *"When you bring up that picture or the _____ (state the situation, event, or stimulus) that triggers you, what would you like to believe about yourself now?"*

_____

Validity of Cognition (VoC)

Say, *"When you think of the _____ (state the situation, event, stimulus, or picture that triggers), how true do those words ____ (clinician repeats the positive cognition) feel to you now on a scale of 1 to 7, where 1 feels completely false and 7 feels completely true?"*

1   2   3   4   5   6   7
(completely false)   (completely true)

Sometimes, it is necessary to explain further.

Say, *"Remember, sometimes we know something with our head, but it feels different in our gut. In this case, what is the gut-level feeling of the truth of _____ (clinician state the positive cognition), from 1 (completely false) to 7 (completely true)?"*

1   2   3   4   5   6   7
(completely false)   (completely true)

Emotions

Say, *"When you bring up the picture (or state the situation, event, or stimulus) that triggers you and those words ____ (clinician states the negative cognition), what emotion do you feel now?"*

_____

Subjective Units of Disturbance (SUD)

Say, *"On a scale of 0 to 10, where 0 is no disturbance or neutral and 10 is the highest disturbance you can imagine, how disturbing does it feel now?"*

0   1   2   3   4   5   6   7   8   9   10
(no disturbance)   (highest disturbance)

Location of Body Sensation

Say, *"Where do you feel it (the disturbance) in your body?"*

_____

Continue to process the triggers according the Standard EMDR Protocol.

Future Template Worksheet (Shapiro, 2006)

The future template is the third prong in the Standard EMDR Protocol. Work with the future template occurs after the earlier memories and present triggers are adequately resolved and the client is ready to make new choices in the future concerning their issue(s). The purpose of it is to address any residual avoidance, any need for further issues of adaptation, to help with incorporating any new information, and to allow for the actualization of client goals. It is another place, in this comprehensive protocol, to catch any fears, negative beliefs, inappropriate responses, and so forth, to reprocess them and also to make sure that the new feelings and behavior can generalize into the clients' day-to-day lives.

There are two basic future templates:

1. Anticipatory Anxiety
   Anticipatory anxiety needs to be addressed with a full assessment (Phase 3) of the future situation.
2. Skills Building and Imaginal Rehearsal
   These do not need a full assessment of target and can begin directly with "running a movie."

Future Template Script
(Shapiro, 2001, pp. 210–214, 2006, pp. 51–53)

Check the Significant People and Situations of the Presenting Issues for any Type of Distress

It is helpful to check to see if all the material concerning the issue upon which the client has worked is resolved or if there is more material that has escaped detection so far. The Future Template is another place to find if there is more material that needs reprocessing.

Significant People

When the client's work has focused on a significant person, ask the following:

Say, *"Imagine yourself encountering that person in the future* _____ (suggest a place that the client might see this person). *What do you notice?"*

_____

_____

Watch the client's reaction to see if more work is necessary. If a client describes a negative feeling in connection with this person, check to see if it is reality based.

Say, *"Is* _____ (state the person's name) *likely to act* _____ (state the client's concern)?"

_____

_____

If the negative feeling is not matching the current reality, say the following:

Say, *"What do you think makes you have negative feelings toward* _____ (state the person in question)?"

_____

_____

If the client is unsure, use the Float-Back or Affect Scan to see what other earlier material may still be active.

If the negative feelings are appropriate, it is important to reevaluate the clusters of events concerning this person and access and reprocess any remaining maladaptive memories. (See Past Memory Worksheet.)

Significant Situations

It is important to have the client imagine being in significant situations in the future; this is another way of accessing material that may not have been processed.

> Say, *"Imagine a videotape or film of how* _____ (state current situation client is working on) *and how it would evolve* _____ (state appropriate time frame) *in the future. When you have done that let me know what you have noticed."*

_____

_____

If there is no disturbance, reinforce the positive experience.

Say, *"Go with that."*

Do BLS.

Reinforce the PC with the future situation with BLS as it continues the positive associations. For further work in the future, see below.

If there is a disturbance, assess what the client needs: more education, modeling of appropriate behavior, or more past memories for reprocessing.

> Say, *"On a scale of 0 to 10, where 0 is no disturbance or neutral and 10 is the highest disturbance you can imagine, how disturbing does it feel now?"*

0	1	2	3	4	5	6	7	8	9	10
(no disturbance)										(highest disturbance)

Anticipatory Anxiety

When the SUD is above 4, or when the Desensitization Phase is not brief, the clinician should look for a present trigger and its associated symptom and develop another Targeting Sequence Plan using the Three-Pronged Protocol. (See worksheets on Past Memories and Present Triggers.)

When there is anticipatory anxiety at a SUD level of no more than 3 to 4 maximum, it is possible to proceed with reprocessing using the future template. The desensitization phase should be quite brief.

> Say, *"What happens when you think of* _____ (state the client's anticipatory anxiety or issue)?"

_____

_____

_____

> Or say, *"When you think of* _____ (state the client's anticipatory anxiety or issue), *what do you get?"*

_____

_____

_____

Picture

Say, "What picture represents the entire _____ (state the client's anticipatory anxiety or issue)?"

_____
_____
_____

If there are many choices or if the client becomes confused, the clinician assists by asking the following:

Say, "What picture represents the most traumatic part of _____ (state the client's anticipatory anxiety or issue)?"

_____
_____
_____

Negative Cognition (NC)

Say, "What words best go with the picture that express your negative belief about yourself now?"

_____
_____

Positive Cognition (PC)

Say, "When you bring up that picture or _____ (state the client's anticipatory anxiety or issue), what would you like to believe about yourself now?"

_____
_____

Validity of Cognition (VoC)

Say, "When you think of _____ (state the client's anticipatory anxiety or issue) or picture, how true do those words _____ (clinician repeats the positive cognition) feel to you now on a scale of 1 to 7, where 1 feels completely false and 7 feels completely true?"

1   2   3   4   5   6   7
(completely false)   (completely true)

Emotions

Say, "When you bring up the picture or _____ (state the client's anticipatory anxiety or issue) and those words _____ (clinician states the negative cognition), what emotion do you feel now?"

_____

Subjective Units of Disturbance (SUD)

Say, "On a scale of 0 to 10, where 0 is no disturbance or neutral and 10 is the highest disturbance you can imagine, how disturbing does it feel now?"

0   1   2   3   4   5   6   7   8   9   10
(no disturbance)   (highest disturbance)

Location of Body Sensation

Say, "*Where do you feel it* (the disturbance) *in your body?*"

___

Phase 4: Desensitization

To begin, say the following:

Say, "*Now remember, it is your own brain that is doing the healing and you are the one in control. I will ask you to mentally focus on the target and to follow my fingers* (or any other BLS you are using). *Just let whatever happens, happen, and we will talk at the end of the set. Just tell me what comes up, and don't discard anything as unimportant. Any new information that comes to mind is connected in some way. If you want to stop, just raise your hand.*"

Then say, "*Bring up the picture and the words* ____ (clinician repeats the NC) *and notice where you feel it in your body. Now, follow my fingers with your eyes* (or other BLS)."

Continue with the Desensitization Phase until the SUD = 0 and the VoC = 7.

Phase 5: Installation

Say, "*How does* ____ (repeat the PC) *sound?*"

___

Say, "*Do the words* ____ (repeat the PC) *still fit, or is there another positive statement that feels better?*"

___

If the client accepts the original positive cognition, the clinician should ask for a VoC rating to see if it has improved.

Say, "*As you think of the incident, how do the words feel, from 1* (completely false) *to 7* (completely true)*?*"

0   1   2   3   4   5   6   7   8   9   10
(no disturbance)   (highest disturbance)

Say, "*Think of the event and hold it together with the words* ____ (repeat the PC)."

Do a long set of BLS to see if there is more processing to be done.

Phase 6: Body Scan

Say, "*Close your eyes and keep in mind the original memory and the positive cognition. Then bring your attention to the different parts of your body, starting with your head and working downward. Any place you find any tension, tightness, or unusual sensation, tell me.*"

___

___

Make sure that this anticipatory anxiety is fully processed before returning to the Future Template.

The Future Template for appropriate future interaction is an expansion of the Installation Phase; instead of linking the positive cognition with the past memory or trigger, the PC is linked to the future issues. Once the client's work has been checked and the other known issues in the past and present have been resolved, each client has the choice to do a more formal future template installation. The first option is to work with the situation or issue as an image.

Image as Future Template: Imagining Positive Outcomes

Imagining positive outcomes seems to assist the learning process. In this way, clients learn to enhance optimal behaviors, to connect them with a positive cognition, and to support generalization. The assimilation of this new behavior and thought is supported by the use of bilateral stimulation (BLS) into a positive way to act in the future.

Say, *"I would like you to imagine yourself coping effectively with or in* _____ (state the goal) *in the future. With the positive belief* _____ (state the positive belief) *and your new sense of* _____ (state the quality: i.e., strength, clarity, confidence, calm), *imagine stepping into this scene. Notice what you see and how you are handling the situation. Notice what you are thinking, feeling, and experiencing in your body."*

_____
_____
_____

Again, here is the opportunity to catch any disturbance that may have been missed.

Say, *"Are there any blocks, anxieties, or fears that arise as you think about this future scene?"*

_____
_____
_____

If yes, say the following:

Say, *"Then focus on these blocks and follow my fingers* (or any other BLS)."

Say, *"What do you get now?"*

_____
_____
_____

If the blocks do not resolve quickly, evaluate if the client needs any new information, resources, or skills to be able to comfortably visualize the future coping scene. Introduce needed information or skills.

Say, *"What would you need to feel confident in handling the situation?"*

_____
_____

Or say, *"What is missing from your handling of this situation?"*

_____
_____

If the block still does not resolve and the client is unable to visualize the future scene with confidence and clarity, use direct questions, the Affect Scan, or the Float-Back Technique to identify old targets related to blocks, anxieties, or fears. Remember, the point of the Three-Prong Protocol is not only to reinforce positive feelings and behavior in the future but again to catch any unresolved material that may be getting in the way of an adaptive resolution of the issue(s). Use the Standard EMDR Protocol to address these targets before proceeding with the template (see Worksheets in this appendix).

If there are no apparent blocks and the client is able to visualize the future scene with confidence and clarity, say the following:

Say, *"Please focus on the image, the positive belief, and the sensations associated with this future scene and follow my fingers* (or any other BLS).*"*

_____

_____

Process and reinforce the positive associations with BLS. Do several sets until the future template is sufficiently strengthened.

Say, *"Go with that."*

_____

Then say, *"Close your eyes and keep in mind the image of the future and the positive cognition. Then bring your attention to the different parts of your body, starting with your head and working downward. Any place you find any tension, tightness, or unusual sensation, tell me."*

_____

If any sensation is reported, do BLS.

Say, *"Go with that."*

If it is a positive or comfortable sensation, do BLS to strengthen the positive feelings.

Say, *"Go with that."*

If a sensation of discomfort is reported, reprocess until the discomfort subsides.

Say, *"Go with that."*

When the discomfort subsides, check the VoC.

Say, *"When you think of the incident* (or picture) *how true do those words ____* (clinician repeats the positive cognition) *feel to you now on a scale of 1 to 7, where 1 feels completely false and 7 feels completely true?"*

    1   2   3   4   5   6   7
(completely false)   (completely true)

Continue to use BLS until reaching the VoC = 7 or there is an ecological resolution. When the image as future template is clear and the PC true, move on to the movie as future template.

Movie as Future Template or Imaginal Rehearsing

During this next level of future template, clients are asked to move from imagining this one scene or snapshot to imagining a movie about coping in the future, with a beginning, middle, and end. Encourage clients to imagine themselves coping effectively in the face of specific challenges, triggers, or snafus. Therapists can make some suggestions in order to help inoculate clients with future problems. It is helpful to use this type of future template after clients have received needed education concerning social skills and customs, assertiveness, and any other newly learned skills.

Say, *"This time, I'd like you to close your eyes and play a movie, imagining yourself coping effectively with or in _____ (state where client will be) in the future. With the new positive belief ___ (state positive belief) and your new sense of ____ (strength, clarity, confidence, calm), imagine stepping into the future. Imagine yourself coping with ANY challenges that come your way. Make sure that this movie has a beginning, middle, and end. Notice what you are seeing, thinking, feeling, and experiencing in your body. Let me know if you hit any blocks. If you do, just open your eyes and let me know. If you don't hit any blocks, let me know when you have viewed the whole movie."*

_____

_____

If the client hits blocks, address as above with BLS until the disturbance dissipates.

Say, *"Go with that."*

If the material does not shift, use interweaves, new skills, information, resources, direct questions, and any other ways to help clients access information that will allow them to move on. If these options are not successful, usually it means that there is earlier material still unprocessed; the Float-Back and Affect Scan are helpful in these cases to access the material that keeps the client stuck.

If clients are able to play the movie from start to finish with a sense of confidence and satisfaction, ask them to play the movie one more time from beginning to end and introduce BLS.

Say, *"Okay, play the movie one more time from beginning to end. Go with that."*

Use BLS.

In a sense, you are installing this movie as a future template.

After clients have fully processed their issue(s), they might want to work on other positive templates for the future in other areas of their lives using the above future templates.

Appendix B: EMDR Worldwide Associations and Other Resources

In the Beginning

The EMDR Institute

Web site: (http://www.emdr.com/)
Contact Person: Robbie Dunton (rdunton@emdr.com)

EMDR Worldwide Associations Contact Information

Africa

Algeria
Contact Person: Mohamed Chakali (chakmed@yahoo.com)

Cameroon
Contact Person: Michelle Depré (emdrcameroun@gmail.com)

Ethiopia
Contact Person: Hiwot Moges (hiwot.moges@gmail.com)
Dorothy Ashman (dorothy.ashman@gmail.com)

Kenya
Association: EMDR Kenya (http://emdrkenya.org)

South Africa
Association: EMDR South Africa/Africa
Contact Person: Reyhana Seedat (rravat@iafrica.com)

Zambia
Contact Person: Sue Gibbons (suegibbonsnow@yahoo.co.uk)
Jack McCarthy (jackmcc5@aol.com)

Asia

EMDR Asia Association: An association of Asian National EMDR Associations (http://www.emdr-asia.org)

Australia
Association: EMDR Association of Australia (http://emdraa.org)

Bangladesh
Contact Person: Shamim Karim (shamim.karim@gmail.com)

Cambodia
Association: EMDR Cambodia Association (http://emdrcambodia.org/)
Contact Person: Bunna Phoeun (bunnasyeng@gmail.com)

China—Mainland
Association: China EMDR (www.emdr.org.cn)
Contact Persons: Jinsong Zhang (zhangjsk@yahoo.com)
Lu Qui-Yun (lvquiyun@263.net)

Hong Kong
Association: The EMDR Association of Hong Kong (http://hkemdr.org)

India
Association: EMDR India (www.emdrindia.org)

Indonesia
Association: EMDR Indonesia (http://www.emdrindonesia.org)

Japan
Association: Japan EMDR Association (http://www.emdr.jp)

Korea
Association: Korean EMDR Association [KEMDRA] (http://emdrkorea.com/fine/)

New Zealand
Association: EMDR New Zealand Association
Contact Person: Astrid Katzur (Astrid.Katzur@emdrnz.org.nz)

Pakistan
Association: EMDR Pakistan (http://emdrpakistan.wordpress.com)

Philippines
Contact Person: Lourdes Medina (lcm50us@yahoo.com)

Singapore
Association: EMDR Singapore (http://www.emdr.sg)

Sri Lanka
Association: Sri Lanka EMDR Association (SEA)
Contact Person: Sr. Janet Nethisinghe (jnethisinghe@yahoo.ca)

Taiwan
Association: Taiwan EMDR Association [TEMDRA] (http://www.temdra.org.tw)

Thailand
Association: EMDR Thailand (http://www.emdrthailand.com)

Vietnam
Contact Person: Dr. Carl Sternberg (pv.carl@gmail.com) Ho Chi Minh City

Europe

EMDR Europe Association: An association of European National EMDR Associations (www.emdr-europe.org)

Austria
Association: EMDR-Netzwerk Osterreich (http://www.emdr-netzwerk.at/)

Belgium
Association: EMDR-Belgium (http://www.emdr-belgium.be)

Denmark
Association: EMDR Danmark (http://www.emdr.dk/)

Finland
Association: Suomen EMDR-Yhdistys (http://www.emdr.fi)

France
Association: Association EMDR France (http://www.emdr-france.org/)

Germany
EMDRIA Deutschland e.V. (http://www.emdria.de)

Greece
Association: EMDR Greece (http://www.emdr.gr/)

Ireland
Association: EMDR UK & Ireland (http://www.emdrassociation.org.uk)

Israel
Association: EMDR-IS (http://www.emdr.org.il)

Italy
Association: EMDR Italie (http://www.emdritalia.it)

Netherlands
Association: Vereniging EMDR Nederland (http://www.emdr.nl)

Norway
Association: EMDR Norge (http://www.emdrnorge.com/)

Poland
Association: PTT EMDR (http://www.emdr.org.pl)

Portugal
Association: EMDR Portugal (http://www.emdrportugal.com)

Serbia
Association: EMDR Serbia (http://www.emdr-se-europe.org)

Slovakia
Contact: Daniel Ralaus (ralaus@hotmail.com)

Spain
Association: Associatión: EMDR-España (www.emdr-es.org)

Sweden
Association: EMDR Sverige (http://www.emdr.se/)

Switzerland
Association: EMDR Schweiz-Suisse-Svizzera-Switzerland (http://www.emdr-schweiz.ch)

Turkey
Association: EMDR Derneği (http://www.emdr-tr.org)

United Kingdom and Ireland
Association: EMDR UK & Ireland (http://www.emdrassociation.org.uk)

EMDR Iberoamérica

EMDR Iberoamérica: An association of South and Central America National EMDR Associations (www.emdriberoamerica.org)

Argentina
Association: EMDR Iberoamérica Argentina (http://www.emdribargentina.org)

Brazil
Association: EMDR Brasil (http://www.emdr.org.br)

Chile
Association: EMDR Chile (http://www.emdrchile.cl)

Colombia
Association: EMDR-IBA Colombia (http://emdrcolombia.com)

Costa Rica
Association: EMDR Costa Rica (http://emdrcostarica.wordpess.com)

Cuba
Contact: Alexis Lorenzo Ruiz (alexis.lorenzo@psico.uh.cu)

Ecuador
Association: EMDR Iberoamérica Ecuador (http://emdrecuador.org)

Guatemala
Association: EMDR Guatemala (http://emdrguatemala.org)
Contact: Ligia Barascout (ligiabps@yahoo.com)

Haiti
Contact: Myrtho Marra Chilosi (emdrhaiti2011@yahoo.fr)

Mexico
Association: EMDR Mexico (http://www.emdrmexico.org)

Panama
Association: EMDR Panama (http://emdribapanama.org/)

Puerto Rico
Association: EMDR Iberoamérica Puerto Rico (http://www.emdribappuertorico.org/)

Uruguay
Association: EMDR Uruguay (http://emdruru.guay.org.uy)

Venezuela
Contact: Deglya Camero de Salazar (deglyac@gmail.com)

North America

Canada
Association: EMDR Canada (http://www.emdrcanada.org)

United States
Association: EMDR International Association (http://emdria.org)

Members of EMDRIA Outside the United States

Iraq
Contact Person: Mona Zaghrout (monazag12@yahoo.com; mzaghrout@ejymca.org)

Lebanon
Association: EMDR Lebanon Association
Contact Person: Lina Ibrahin (lina_f_ibrahim@hotmail.com)

Palestine
Contact Person: Mona Zaghrout (monazag12@yahoo.com; mzaghrout@ejymca.org)

Related EMDR Humanitarian Associations

Asia

Japan
Association: JEMDRA-HAP (http://hap.emdr.jp/)

Europe

HAP-Europe
Association: HAP-Europe (http://www.emdr-europe.org)

France
Association: HAP-France (http://www. http://hap-france.blogspot.fr)

Germany
Association: Trauma Aid (http://www.trauma-aid.org)

Spain
Association: HAP-España (http://www.emdr-es.org)

Switzerland
Association: HAP-Schweiz-Suisse-Svizzera-Switzerland (http://www.emdrschweiz.ch)

Turkey
Association: EMDR-HAP Turkey (www.emdr-tr.com)
Contact Person: Senel Karaman (senelkaraman@gmail.com)

United Kingdom and Ireland
Association: HAP UK & Ireland (www.hapuk.org)

Ibero-America

Argentina
Association: EMDR-Programa de Programa de Ayuda Humanitaria–Argentina
Email: emdrasistenciahumanitaria@fibertel.com.ar(Web site under construction at same address)

Iberoamerica
EMDR Iberoamerica (http://emdriberoamerica.org/progamaayudahumanitaria.html/)

Mexico
Asociacion Mexicana para Ayuda Mental en Crisis A.C. (http://www.amamecrisis.com.mx)

North America

United States
EMDR Humanitarian Assistance Program [EMDR-HAP] (http://www.emdrhap.org)

The Francine Shapiro Library

Francine Shapiro Library's EMDR Bibliography (http://library.nku.edu/)

EMDR Journals and E-Journals

The Journal of EMDR Practice and Research—The official publication of the EMDR International Association (http://www.springerpub.com/emdr)

EMDR-IS Electronic Journal (http://www.emdr.org.il)

Related EMDR Information

EMDR Network (http://www.emdrnetwork.org)

EMDR Research Foundation (http://www.emdrresearch.org)

Related Traumatology Information

American Red Cross (www.redcross.org)

The Australian Trauma Web (http://welcome.to/ptsd)David Baldwin's Trauma Pages (http://www.trauma-pages.com)

Children and War (http://www.childrenandwar.org)

European Federation of Psychologists Associations Task Force on Disaster Psychology [EFPA] (http://www.disaster.efpa.eu)

European Society for Traumatic Stress Studies (http://www.estss.org)

Give an Hour (www.giveanhour.org/)

International Society for the Study of Trauma and Dissociation (http://www.isst-d.org)

The International Critical Incident Stress Foundation (http://www.icisf.org)

National Center for PTSD (http://www.ptsd.va.gov)

National Institute of Mental Health (http://www.nimh.nih.gov/health/topics/post-traumatic-stress-disorder-ptsd/index.shtml)

United States National Center for Posttraumatic Stress Disorder (http://www.ncptsd.va.gov/ncmain/index.jsp)

Wounded Warrior Project (www.woundedwarriorproject.org)

References and Bibliography

Adler-Tapia, A. (2012). *Child psychotherapy: Integrating developmental theory into clinical practice*. New York, NY: Springer Publishing.

Adúriz, M. E., Knopfler, C., & Bluthgen, C. (2009). Helping child flood victims using group EMDR intervention in Argentina: Treatment outcome and gender differences. *International Journal of Stress Management, 16(2)*, 138–153.

Alter-Reid, K., Evans, S., & Schaefer, S. (2010, October). *Therapy for Therapists Project: Impact of intensive EMDR treatment post-Katrina*. Paper presented at the EMDRIA Conference, Minneapolis, MN.

American Psychiatric Association. (2000). *Diagnostic and statistical manual of mental disorders-fourth edition text revision*. Washington, DC: Author.

American Psychiatric Association. (2004a). *Diagnostic and statistical manual for mental disorders. DSM-IV-TR* (4th ed., rev. text). Washington, DC: Author.

American Psychiatric Association. (2004b). *Practice Guideline for the treatment of patients with acute stress disorder and post-traumatic stress disorder*. Arlington, VA: Author.

Anderson, M. B., Brown, D., & Jean, I. (2012). *Time to listen, hearing people on the receiving end of international aid*. Cambridge, MA: CDA Collaborative Learning Projects.

Andrews, B., Brewin, C. R., Philpott, R., & Stewart, L. (2007). Delayed-onset posttraumatic stress disorder: A systematic review of the evidence. *American Journal of Psychiatry, 164(9)*, 1319–1326.

Armstrong, K., O'Callahan, W., Marmar, C. R. (1991). Debriefing Red Cross Disaster Personnel: The multiple stressor debriefing model. *Journal of Traumatic Stress 4*, 581–593.

Artigas, L., & Jarero, I. (2009). The butterfly hug. In M. Luber (Ed.) *Eye movement desensitization and reprocessing (EMDR) scripted protocols: Special populations* (pp. 5–7). New York, NY: Springer.

Artigas, L., Jarero, I., Alcalá, N., & Lopez-Cano, T. (2009). The EMDR integrative group treatment protocol (IGTP). In M. Luber (Ed.) *Eye movement desensitization and reprocessing (EMDR) scripted protocols: Basic and special situations* (pp. 279–288). New York, NY: Springer.

Artigas, L., Jarero, I., Mauer, M., López Cano, T., & Alcalá, N. (2000, September). *EMDR and traumatic stress after natural disasters: Integrative treatment protocol and the butterfly hug*. Poster presented at the EMDRIA Conference, Toronto, ON, Canada.

Artwohl, A. (2002). Perceptual and memory distortions in officer involved shootings. *FBI Law Enforcement Bulletin, 10*, 18–24.

Arvay, M. J., & Uhlemann, M. R. (1996). Counsellor stress in the field of trauma: A preliminary study. *Canadian Journal of Counselling, 30*, 193–121.

Ayalon, O. (1976). *Rescue! An emergency handbook*. Haifa, Israel: University of Haifa Press.

Ayalon, O., Lahad, M., & Cohen, A. (1999). *Community Stress Prevention*. Vol 3,4 1999. The Community Stress Prevention Center, Jerusalem Ministry of Education, Kiryat Shmona, Israel.

Ayalon, O. (2003). The HANDS project: Helpers assisting natural disaster survivors. *Community Stress Prevention Centre, 5*, 127–135.

Bar-Sade, E. (2003a). *Early trauma: Revisited and revised through EMDR, the narrative story and the implementation of attachment theory*. Paper presented at the EMDR European Annual Conference, Rome.

Bar-Sade, E. (2003b). *EMDR and children*. The International Trauma Conference, Jerusalem.

Bar-Sade, E. (2005a). *"Attachment cues" as resources in affect regulation enhancement in children's EMDR Processing*. EMDR European Conference, Stockholm.

Bar-Sade, E. (2005b). EMDR and the challenge of working with children. *EMDR-Israel E-Journal*, www.emdr.org.il (Hebrew).

Bar-Sade, E. (2005c). EMDR with children. *EMDR-Israel E-Journal*, www.emdr.org.il (Hebrew).

Baruch, Y. (2009, January). *Mental health assistance in national emergencies: Initial phase*. Paper presented at the International Conference on Crisis as an Opportunity: Organizational and Professional Responses to Disaster, Ben-Gurion University of the Negev, Beer-Sheva, Israel.

Baum, N. (2010). Shared traumatic reality in communal disasters: Towards a conceptualization. *Psychotherapy Theory, Research, Practice, Training, 47(2)*, 249–259.

Beaton, R. D., & Murphy, S. A. (1995). Working with people in crisis: Research implications. In C. R. Figley (Ed.), *Compassion fatigue: Coping with secondary traumatic stress disorder in those who treat the traumatized* (pp. 51–81). New York, NY: Brunner/Mazel.

Beck, A. T., Ward, C., & Mendelson, M. (1961). Beck Depression Inventory (BDI). *Archives for General Psychiatry*, 4(6), 561–571.

Beebe, G. W., & Appel, J. W. (1958). Variation in psychological tolerance to ground combat in World War II. Washington, DC: National Academy of Sciences.

Birnbaum, A. (2005a, February). *Group EMDR with children and families in South Thailand post-tsunami*. Invited presentation at Bangkok Children's Hospital, Bangkok, Thailand.

Birnbaum, A. (2005b, February). *Group EMDR with children and families following the tsunami in Thailand*. Invited presentation at the EMDR-Israel Humanitarian Assistance Program Conference, Ra'anana, Israel.

Birnbaum, A. (2006, July). *Group EMDR: Theory and practice*. Invited presentation at the EMDR-Israel Humanitarian Assistance Program Conference, Netanya, Israel.

Birnbaum, A. (2007, February). *Group EMDR in critical incident stress debriefing with IDF casualty notification officers: A pilot study*. Invited presentation at the EMDR-Israel Conference on EMDR in the Second Lebanese War, Netanya, Israel.

Bleich, A., Gelkopf, M., & Solomon, Z. (2003). Exposure to terrorism, stress related mental health symptoms, and coping behaviours among a nationally representative sample in Israel. *JAMA*, 290, 612–620.

Blore, D. C. (2009). Blind to therapist protocol. In M. Luber (Ed.), *Eye movement desensitization and reprocessing (EMDR) scripted protocols: Basics and special situations* (chap. 25). New York, NY: Springer.

Blore, D. C. (1997). Reflections on "A day when the whole world seemed to be darkened" changes. *International Journal of Psychology and Psychotherapy, 15(2)*, 89–95.

Blore, D., Holmshaw, E. M., Swift, A., Standart, S., & Fish, D. M. (2013). The development and uses of the "Blind to Therapist" EMDR Protocol. *Journal Of EMDR Practice and Research, 7*, 2, pp. 95–105.

Boel, J. (1999). The butterfly hug. *EMDRIA Newsletter*, 4(4), 11–13.

Brewin, C. R., Rose, S., Andrews, B., Green, J., Turner, S., & Foa, E. (2002). Brief screening instrument for post-traumatic stress disorder. *British Journal of Psychiatry, 181*, 158–162.

Briere, J., & Scott, C. (2006). *Principles of trauma therapy: A guide to symptoms, evaluation and treatment*. Thousand Oaks, CA: Sage.

Bryant, R. A. (2007). Early intervention for post-traumatic stress disorder. *Early Intervention in Psychiatry, 1*, 19–26.

Bryant, R. A., & Harvey, A. G. (2000). *Acute stress disorder: A handbook of theory, assessment, and treatment*. Washington, DC: American Psychological Association.

Buchanan, M., Anderson, J., Uhlemann, M., & Horwitz, E. (2006, December). Secondary traumatic stress: An investigation of Canadian mental health workers. *Traumatology, 12,* 272–281.

Carlson, E, B., & Putnam, F. W. (1992). *Manual for the dissociative experiences scale.* Lutherville, MD: Sidran Foundation.

Cemalovic, A. (1997). *A saga of Sarajevo children: Coping with life under siege.* Stockholm, Sweden: KTH Hogskoletryckeriet.

Chemtob, C. M., & Dutch, H. (2006). *Bi-national trauma response: Building psychosocial resiliency in Sri Lanka [Evaluation report].* New York, NY: UJA Fed NY.

Chemtob, C. M., Nakashima, J., & Carlson, J. G. (2002). Brief-treatment for elementary school children with disaster-related posttraumatic stress disorder: A field study. *Journal of Clinical Psychology, 58,* 99–112.

Cocco, N., & Sharpe, L. (1993). An auditory variant of eye movement desensitization in a case of childhood post-traumatic stress disorder. *Journal of Behavior Therapy and Experimental Psychiatry, 24, 373–377.*

Connor, K. M., & Davidson, J. R. T. (2001, September). SPRINT: A brief global assessment of post-traumatic stress disorder. *International Clinical Psychopharmacology, 16(5),* 279–284.

Crespo, M., & Gomez, M. M. (2011). *EGEP Evaluación Global del Estrés Postraumático.* Madrid, Spain: TEA Ediciones.

Daniels, N. (2009). Self-care for EMDR practitioners. In M. Luber (Ed.). *Eye movement desensitization and reprocessing (EMDR) Scripted Protocols: Basics and special situations* (pp. 399–400). New York, NY: Springer.

de Roos, C., & van Rood, Y. R. (2009). EMDR in the treatment of medically unexplained symptoms: A systematic review. *Journal of EMDR Practice and Research, 3,* 248–263.

Department of the Army. (2006). *Combat and operational stress control: Field manual No. 4-02.51 (FM 8 51).* Washington, DC: Headquarters, Department of the Army.

Department of Veteran's Affairs & Department of Defense. (2009). *VA/DoD evidence based clinical practice guideline for management of concussion/mild traumatic brain injury.* Washington, DC: The Office of Quality and Performance & Quality Management Directorate, United States Army MEDCOM, VA.

Department of Veteran's Affairs & Department of Defense. (2010). *VA/DoD clinical practice guideline for the management of post-traumatic stress* (Office of Quality and Performance Publication 10Q-CPG/PTSD-10). Washington, DC: Veterans Health Administration, Department of Veterans Affairs and Health Affairs, Department of Defense. Retrieved from www.healthquality.va.gov/ptsd/ptsd_full.pdf

Derogatis, L. R. (1983). *SCL-90-R administration, scoring & procedures manual-II* (pp. 14–15). Towson, MD: Clinical Psychometric Research.

Derogatis, L. R. (1993). *Brief Symptom Inventory: Administration, scoring, and procedures manual.* Minneapolis, MN: National Computer Systems.

Dyregov, A. (1989). Caring for helpers in disaster situations: Psychological debriefings. *Disaster Management, 2,* 25–30.

Elliott, D. M., & Briere, J. (1992). Sexual abuse trauma among professional women: Validating the Trauma Symptom Checklist-40 (TSC-40). *Child Abuse & Neglect, 16(3),* 391–398.

Emanuel, Y. (2006, August). Integrating EMDR and a narrative approach in treatment of complex trauma. *EMDR-Israel E-Journal,* www.emdr.org.il (Hebrew).

Errebo, N., Knipe, J., Forte, K., Karlin, V., & Altayli, B. (2008). EMDR-HAP Training in Sri Lanka following 2004 tsunami. *Journal of EMDR Practice & Research, 2(2),* 124–139.

Escudero, A. (2003). *Healing by thinking. Noesitherapy (Biological basis)* (4th ed.). Impreso en Signo Grafico: Valencia, Espana (web-site: http://dr.escudero.com/comprar.html.)

Etherington, K. (2009). Supervising helpers who work with the trauma of sexual abuse. *British Journal of Guidance and Counselling, 37(2),* 179–194.

Everly, G. S., Boyle, S. & Lating. J. (1999). The effectiveness of psychological debriefing in vicarious trauma: A meta-analysis. *Stress Medicine, 15,* 229–233.

Everly, G. S., Jr., & Mitchell, J. T. (2008). *Integrative crisis intervention and disaster mental health.* Ellicott City, MD: Chevron.

Fernandez, I. (2002, Dicembre). I disturbi post-traumatici da stress, fattori di rischio, aspetti diagnostici e trattamento con l'EMDR [The post-traumatic stress disorder factors of risk, diagnostic aspects and treatment with EMDR]. Rivista Scientifica di Psicologia, Sommario 01, 15–24.

Fernandez, I., Gallinari, E., & Lorenzetti, A. (2004). A school-based intervention for children who witnessed the Pirelli building airplane crash in Milan, Italy. *Journal of Brief Therapy, 2*, 129–136.

Figley, C. R. (Ed.). (1995). *Compassion fatigue: Coping with secondary traumatic stress disorder in those who treat the traumatized.* New York, NY: Bruner/Mazel.

Figley, C. R. (2002). *Treating compassion fatigue.* New York, NY: Brunner-Rutledge.

Figley, C. R., & Kleber, R. J. (1995). Beyond the "victim": Secondary traumatic stress. In R. J. Kleber, C.R. Figley, & B. P. R. Gersons (Eds.), *Beyond trauma: Cultural and societal dynamics* (pp. 75–98). New York, NY: Plenum Press.

Foa, E. B., Cashman, L., Jaycox, L., & Perry, K. (1997). The validation of a self-report measure of posttraumatic stress disorder: The Posttraumatic Diagnostic Scale. *Psychological Assessment, 9*(4), 445–451.

Foa, E. B., & Riggs, D. S. (1994). Posttraumatic stress disorder and rape. In R. S. Pynoos (Ed.), *Posttraumatic stress disorder: A clinical review* (pp. 133–163). Baltimore, MD: Sidran Press.

Foa, E. B., Riggs, D. S., Dancu, C. V., & Rothbaum, B. O. (1993). Reliability and validity of a brief instrument for assessing post-traumatic stress disorder. *Journal of Traumatic Stress, 6*(4), 459–473.

French, D. P., & Sutton, S. (2010). Reactivity of measurement in health psychology: How much of a problem is it? What can be done about it? *British Journal of Health Psychology, 15*(Pt. 3), 453–468.

Galliano, S., Cervera, M., & Parada, E. (2004). *El CIPR Procesamiento y Recuperación tras Incidentes Críticos.* Retrieved from http://hdl.handle.net/10401/2975

Galliano, S., & Lahad, M. (2002). Debriefing reconsidered. *Counseling and Psychotherapy Journal, 3*(2), 20–21.

Gawrych, A. L. (2010). *PTSD in firefighters and secondary trauma in their wives.* Hempstead, NY: Hofstra University.

Gelbach, R., & Davis, K. (2007). Disaster response: EMDR and family systems therapy under communitywide stress. In F. Shapiro, F. W. Kaslow, & L. Maxfield (Eds.), *Handbook of EMDR and family therapy processes* (pp. 387–406). Hoboken, NJ: Wiley.

Gelinas, D. J. (2003). Integrating EMDR into phase-oriented treatment for trauma. *Journal of Trauma and Dissociation, 4*, 91–135.

Gilbar, O., Plivazky, N., & Gil, S. (2010). Counterfactual thinking, coping strategies, and coping resources as predictors of PTSD diagnosed in physically injured victims of terror attacks. *Journal of Loss and Trauma, 15*, 304–324.

Grainger, R. D., Levin, C., Allen-Byrd, L., Doctor, R. M., & Lee, H. (1997). An empirical evaluation of eye movement desensitization and reprocessing (EMDR) with survivors of a natural disaster. *Journal of Traumatic Stress, 10*, 665–671.

Greenwald, R. (1994). Applying eye movement desensitization and reprocessing to the treatment of traumatized children: Five case studies. *Anxiety Disorders Practice Journal, 1*, 83–97.

Greenwald, R. (1998). Eye movement desensitization and reprocessing (EMDR): New hope for children suffering from trauma and loss. *Clinical Child Psychology and Psychiatry, 3*, 279–287.

Greenwald, R., & Rubin, A. (1999). Brief assessment of children's post-traumatic symptoms: Development and preliminary validation of parent and child scales. *Research on Social Work Practice, 9*, 61–75.

Greenwald, R. (1999). *Eye movement desensitization and reprocessing (EMDR) in child and adolescent psychotherapy.* Northvale, NJ: Jason Aronson Press.

Greenwald, R. (2000). A trauma-focused individual therapy approach for adolescents with conduct disorder. *International Journal of Offender Therapy and Comparative Criminology, 44*, 146–163.

Grenough, M. (2012). *Oasis in the overwhelm.* New Haven, CT: Beaver Hill Press.

Grieger, T. A., Cozza, S. J., Ursano, R. J., Hoge, C., Martinez, P. E., Engel, C. C., & Wain, H. J. (2006). Posttraumatic stress disorder and depression in battle-injured soldiers. *American Journal of Psychiatry, 163*(10), 1777–1783.

Grossman, D. (2007). *On combat: The psychology and physiology of deadly conflict in war and in peace* (2nd ed.). Millstadt, Illinois: PPCT Research.

Herman, J. L. (1992). *Trauma and recovery*. New York, NY: Basic Books.

Hernandez, D. (2002). DRC: District resource center defined. *Insights*. Retrieved from http://www.openinc.org/newsletters/Insights_2002Fall.pdf

Holbrook, T. L., Galarneau, M. R., Dye, J. L., Quinn, K., & Dougherty, A. L. (2010). Morphine use after combat injury in Iraq and post-traumatic stress disorder. *New England Journal of Medicine, 362*, 110–117.

Holgersen, K. H., Klöckner, C. A., Boe, H. J., Weisaeth, L., & Holen, A. (2011). Disaster survivors in their third decade: Trajectories of initial stress responses and long term course of mental health. *Journal of Traumatic Stress, 24*(3), 334–341.

Honig, A., & Roland, J. (1998). Shots fired: Officer involved. *The Police Chief, 65*, 16–19.

Horowitz, M. J. (1979). Psychological response to serious life events. In V. Hamilton & D. M. Warburton (Eds.), *Human stress and cognition* (pp. 235–263). Chichester, England: Wiley.

Horowitz, M. J., Wilner, M., & Alverez, W. (1979). Impact of Events Scale: A measure of subjective stress. *Psychosomatic Medicine, 41*(3), 209–218.

Ironson, G. I., Freund, B., Strauss, J. L., & Williams, J. (2002). A comparison of two treatments for traumatic stress: A pilot study of EMDR and prolonged exposure. *Journal of Clinical Psychology, 58*, 113–128.

Ivar, Pivar (2004). Traumatic grief: Symptomatology and treatment in the Iraq War veteran. In The Department of Veterans' Affairs National Center of PTSD, *Iraq War clinician guide* (2nd ed., pp. 75–78). Department of Veteran's Affairs, National Centre for PTSD.

Jarero, I. (2011). *El Desastre Después del Desastre: ¿Ya pasó lo peor? Revista Iberoamericana de Psicotraumatología y Disociación* (Volumen 1, Número 1). Retrieved from http://revibapst.com/DESASTRE-REVIBA.pdf

Jarero, I., & Artigas, L. (2009). EMDR integrative group treatment protocol. *Journal of EMDR Practice and Research, 3*(4), 287–288.

Jarero, I., Artigas, L., & Hartung, J. (2006). EMDR integrative group treatment protocol: A post-disaster trauma intervention for children and adults. *Traumatology, 12*, 121–129.

Jarero, I., & Artigas, L. (2010). The EMDR integrative group treatment protocol: Application with adults during ongoing geopolitical crisis. *Journal of EMDR Practice and Research, 4*(4), 148–155.

Jarero, I., Artigas, L., & Hartung, J. (2006). EMDR integrative group treatment protocol: A post-disaster trauma intervention for children and adults. *Traumatology, 12*, 121–129.

Jarero, I., Artigas, L., & Luber, M. (2011). The EMDR protocol for recent critical incidents: Application in a disaster mental health continuum of care context. *Journal of EMDR Practice and Research, 5*(3), 82–94.

Jarero, I., Artigas, L., Mauer, M., López Cano, T., & Alcalá, N. (1999, November). *Children's post traumatic stress after natural disasters: Integrative treatment protocol*. Poster presented at the annual meeting of the International Society for Traumatic Stress Studies, Miami, FL.

Jarero, I., Artigas, L., Montero, M. (2008). The EMDR integrative group treatment protocol: Application with child victims of mass disaster. *Journal of EMDR Practice & Research, 2*(2), 97–105.

Jarero, I., & Uribe, S. (2011). The EMDR protocol for recent critical incidents: Brief report of an application in a human massacre situation. *Journal of EMDR Practice and Research, 5*(4), 156–165.

Jarero, I., & Uribe, S. (2012). The EMDR protocol for recent critical incidents: Follow-up report of an application in a human massacre situation. *Journal of EMDR Practice and Research, 6*(2), 50–61.

Jelinek, P., & Burns, R. (2012, January). *Pentagon works on new plan to curb sex assaults*. Retrieved from http://www.huffingtonpost.com/2012/01/ll/marines-urinate-corpses-video-afghanistan_n_1200513.html

Jelinek, P. & Burns, R. (2012, January). Panetta assures Afghans of full probe into video. OnlineAthens (Athens Banner-Herald), (http://onlineathens.com/do/not/override/panel/taxonomy/term/43481/2)

Johnson, K. (1998). *Trauma in the lives of children*. Alameda, CA: Hunter House.

Jones, E., & Wessley, S. (2003). Forward psychiatry in the military: Its origins and effectiveness. *Journal of Traumatic Stress, 16(4)*, 411–419.

Jones, E., & Wessely, S. (2005). *Shell shock to PTSD: Military psychiatry from 1900 to the Gulf War*. New York, NY: Psychology Press.

Jones, R. (1997). Child's reaction to traumatic event scale (CRTES). In J. Wilson & T. Keane (Eds.), *Assessing psychological trauma and PTSD* (pp. 291–348). New York, NY: Guilford Press.

Jones, R. T., Fletcher, K., & Ribbe, D. R. (2004). Child's reaction to traumatic event scale-revised (CRTES-R). In J. Wilson & T. Keane (Eds.), *Assessing psychological trauma and PTSD* (2nd ed., p. 523). New York, NY: Guilford Press.

Kabat-Zinn, J. (2012). *Mindfulness for beginners*. CT: Sounds True.

Kaplan G. (1975). *Support Systems in Times of War, The Individual and the Community in Emergencies*. Hebrew University, Jerusalem (Hebrew)

Klingman, A., & Ayalon, O. (1976). Preparing the education system for emergency. *Israeli Journal of Psychology and Counseling in Education (Chavat Da'at), 15*, 135–148. (Hebrew)

Konuk, E. (2009, June). Mental health response and training program for developing countries: The Turkish model. In G. Zaal (Chair), *Diverse*. Symposium conducted at the annual meeting of the EMDR Europe Association, Amsterdam, the Netherlands.

Konuk, E., Knipe, J., Eke, I., Yuksek, H., Yurtsever, A., & Ostep, S. (2006). The effects of eye movement desensitization and reprocessing (EMDR) therapy on post-traumatic stress disorder in survivors of the 1999 Marmara, Turkey, earthquake. *International Journal of Stress Management, 13(3)*, 291–308. doi:10.1037/1072-5245.13.3.291

Korkmazlar-Oral, U., & Pamuk, S. (2002). Group EMDR with child survivors of the earthquake in Turkey. *Journal of the American Academy of Child and Adolescent Psychiatry, 37*, 47–50.

Korn, D., & Leeds, A. M. (2002). Preliminary evidence of efficacy for EMDR resource development and installation in the stabilization phase of treatment of complex posttraumatic stress disorder. *Journal of Clinical Psychology, 58*, 1465–1487.

Kristal-Andersson, B. (2000). *Psychology of the refugee, the immigrant and their children: Development of a conceptual framework and applications to psychotherapeutic and related support work*. Lund, Sweden: University of Lund Press.

Kutz, I., Dekel, R., Schreiber, S., Resnick, V., Dolberg, O. T., Barkai, G., . . . Bloch, M. (2008, November). *The effect of a single session of EMDR on intrusive distress in acute stress syndromes*. Symposium/panel conducted at the 24th annual meeting of the International Society for Traumatic Stress Studies, Chicago, IL.

L'Abate, L. (2004). *A guide to self-help mental health workbooks for clinicians and researchers*. Binghamton, NY: Haworth.

Lahad, M. (2005, October). *1st report to JDC & UJA Fed NY, on the progress of the Tri National project*. Unpublished manuscript, Community Stress Prevention Center, Kiryat Shmona, Israel.

Lahad, M. (2009). *Lessons learnt from the Tri-National project in Sri Lanka following the 2004 tsunami: Focusing on culturally sensitive issues of mental health and psychosocial support and the management of such a project*. Paper presented at the International Conference on Crisis as an Opportunity: Organizational and Professional Responses to Disaster, Ben-Gurion University of the Negev, Beer-Sheva, Israel.

Lahad, M. (2011). *Lessons learned: What was effective post natural disaster training 5 years after the MT training in Sri Lanka was over (2007) field visit and group interview*. A report submitted to UJA Fed. NY and to ITC.

Lahad, M. (2013). BASIC Ph: The story of coping resources. In M. Lahad, M. Shacham, & O. Ayalon (Eds.), *The "BASIC PH" model of coping and resiliency—Theory, research and cross-cultural application*. London, England: Jessica Kingsley.

Lahad, M., Baruch, Y., Shacham, Y., Niv, S., Rogel, R, Nacasch, N., . . . Leykin, D. (2011). Cultural sensitivity in psychosocial interventions following a disaster: A trinational collaboration in Sri Lanka. In R. Kaufman, R. L. Edwards, J. Mirsky, & A. Avgar (Eds.), *Crisis as an opportunity: Organizational and professional responses to disaster* (pp. 129–154). Lanham, MD: University Press of America.

Lahad, M., & Cohen, A. (1997). *Community stress preventions* (Vols. 1, 2). Kiryat Shmona, Israel: The Community Stress Prevention Center, Jerusalem Ministry of Education.

Lamphear, M. (2010). *Effectiveness of the post critical incident seminar in reducing critical incident stress among law enforcement officers*. Doctoral dissertation, Walden University.

Lande, R. G., Marin, B. A., & Ruzek, J. I. (2004). Substance abuse in the deployment environment. In The Department of Veterans Affairs National Center of PTSD (Eds.), *Iraq War clinician guide* (2nd ed., pp. 79–82). Department of Veterans Affairs, National Center of PTSD. Retrieved from: www.ptsd.va.gov

Lansen, J. (1993). Vicarious traumatization in therapists treating victims of torture and persecution. *Torture*, 3(4), 138–140.

Lansen, J., & Haans, T. (2004). Clinical supervision for trauma therapists. In J. P. Wilson & B. Drozdek (Eds.), *Broken spirits: The treatment of traumatized asylum seekers, refugees, war and torture victims* (pp. 317–354). New York, NY: Brunner-Routledge.

Laub, B. (2001). The healing power of resource connection in the EMDR protocol [Special edition]. *EMDRIA Newsletter*, 21–27.

Laub, B. (2009). Resource connection envelope (RCE) in the EMDR Standard Protocol. In Luber, M. (Ed.), *EMDR Scripted Protocols: Basic and Special Situations (pp. 93–99)*. New York, NY: Springer.

Laub, B., & Bar-Sade, E. (2009). The Imma EMDR group protocol. In M. Luber (Ed.), *Eye movement desensitization and reprocessing (EMDR) scripted protocols: Basic and special situations* (p. 292). New York, NY: Springer.

Laub, B., & Weiner, N. (2007). The pyramid model—Dialectical polarity in therapy. *Journal of Transpersonal Psychology*, 39(2), 199–221.

Laub, B., & Weiner, N. (2011). A developmental/integrative perspective of the recent traumatic episode protocol (R-TEP). *Journal of EMDR Practice and Research*, 5(2), 57–72.

Lee, C., Gavriel, H., Drummond, P., Richards, J., & Greenwald, R. (2002). Treatment of PTSD: Stress inoculation training with prolonged exposure compared to EMDR. *Journal of Clinical Psychology*, 58, 1071–1089.

Leeds, A. M. (2009). *A guide to the standard EMDR protocols for clinicians, supervisors, and consultants*. New York, NY: Springer.

Levine, P. (1997). *Waking the tiger: Healing trauma*. Berkeley, CA: North Atlantic Book.

Leykin, D. (2012, September). *Crisis management in schools (CIMS) preliminary results from a controlled study* [Research report]. Unpublished manuscript, Community Stress Prevention Center, Kiryat Shmona, Israel.

Litz, B. T. (Ed.). (2004). *Early intervention for trauma and traumatic loss*. New York, NY: Guilford Press.

Lovett, J. (1999). *Small wonders: Healing childhood trauma with EMDR*. New York, NY: Free Press.

Luber, M. (2001, December). In the spotlight. Roger Solomon. EMDRIA Newsletter, 6, 4, 20–21.

Laub, B. (2009). Resource Connection Envelope (RCE) in the EMDR standard protocol. In M. Luber (Ed.), *EMDR scripted protocols: Basic and special situations* (pp. 93–99). New York: Springer

Luber, M. (Ed.) (2009a). *Eye movement desensitization and reprocessing (EMDR) scripted protocols: Basics and special situations*. New York, NY: Springer.

Luber, M. (Ed.). (2009b). *Eye movement desensitization and reprocessing (EMDR): Scripted protocols basics and special situations* (pp. 387–392). New York, NY: Springer.

Luber, M. (Ed.). (2009c). *Eye movement desensitization and reprocessing (EMDR): Scripted protocols basics and special situations* (Section, III, pp. 67–106). New York, NY: Springer.

Luber, M. (Scripted by). (2009d). Recent traumatic events protocol. In M. Luber (Ed.), *Eye movement desensitization and reprocessing (EMDR): Scripted protocols basics and special situations* (pp. 387–392). New York, NY: Springer.

Luber, M., & Shapiro, F. (2009). Interview with Francine Shapiro: Historical overview, present issues, and future directions of EMDR. *Journal of EMDR Practice and Research, 3*(4), 217–231.

Ludwig, A., & Ranson, S. (1947). A statistical follow-up of effectiveness of treatment of combat-induced psychiatric casualties: 1. Returns to full combat duty. *Military Surgeon, 100,* 51–62.

Macy, R., Behart, L., Paulson, R., Delman, J., Schmid, L., & Smith, S. F. (2004). Community-based, acute posttraumatic stress management: A description and evaluation of a psychosocial-intervention continuum. *Harvard Review of Psychiatry, 12,* 217–218.

Maguan, S., Lucenko, B. A., Reger, M. A., Gahm, G. A., Litz, B. T., Seal, K. H., . . . Marmar, C. R. (2010). The impact of reported direct and indirect killing on mental health symptoms in Iraq war veterans. *Journal of Traumatic Stress, 23*(1), 86–90.

Maguen, S., Metzler, T., McCaslin, S., Inslicht, S., Henn-Haase, C., Neylan, T., & Marmar, C. (2009). Routine work environment stress and PTSD symptoms in police officers. *Journal of Nervous & Mental Disease, 197*(10), 754–760.

Manfield, P., & Shapiro, F. (2003). The application of EMDR to the treatment of personality disorders. In J. F. Magnavita (Ed.), *Handbook of personality: Theory and practice.* Hoboken, NJ: Wiley.

Marin, P. (1995). *Freedom & its discontents: Reflection on four decades of American moral experience.* South Royalton, VT: Steerforth Press.

Marmar, C. R., Weiss, D. S., & Metzler, T. J. (1996). The Peritraumatic Dissociative Experiences Questionnaire. In J. P. Wilson & C. R. Marmar (Eds.), *Assessing psychological trauma and posttraumatic stress disorder* (pp. 412–428). New York, NY: Guilford Press.

Maslach, C., Jackson, S. E., & Leiter, M. P. (1996). *Maslach Burnout Inventory manual* (3rd ed.). Palo Alto, CA: Consulting Psychologists Press.

Maxfield, L. (2008). EMDR treatment of recent events and community disasters. *Journal of EMDR Practice & Research, 2*(2), 74–78.

Maxfield, L. (2009). Twenty years of EMDR. *Journal of EMDR Practice and Research, 3*(4), 211–216.

Maxfield, L., Melnyk, W. T., & Hayman, C. A. G. (2008). A working memory explanation for the effects of eye movements in EMDR. *Journal of EMDR Practice and Research, 2*(4), 247–261.

McCann, I. L., & Pearlman, L. A. (1990). Vicarious traumatization: A contextual model for understanding the effects of trauma on helpers. *Journal of Traumatic Stress, 3*(1), 131–149.

McCullough, L. (2002). Exploring change mechanisms in EMDR applied to "small t-trauma" in short term dynamic psychotherapy: Research questions and speculations. *Journal of Clinical Psychology, 58,* 1465–1487.

McFarlane, A. C. (2010). The long-term costs of traumatic stress: Intertwined physical and psychological consequences. *World Psychiatry, 9,* 3–10.

McNally, V. J., & Solomon, R. M. (1999, February). The FBI's critical incident stress management program. *FBI Law Enforcement Bulletin,* pp. 20–26.

Mehrotra, S. (1996). *EMDR an integrated approach to psychotherapy.* Paper presented at the Bombay Psychological Association Annual Conference, Bombay, India.

Mehrotra, S. (2008, June). *EMDR in India.* Keynote and paper presented at the 9th EMDR European Conference, London.

Mehrotra, S., & Geng, W. (2011, February). EMDR in India. *Journal of Xihua University (Philosophy & Social Sciences).* doi:CNKI:SUN:CDSF.0.2011-02-000

Meichenbaum, D. (1994). *A clinical handbook/practical therapist manual for assessing and treating adults with post-traumatic stress disorder (PTSD).* Waterloo, Canada: Institute Press.

Melville, A. (2003, April). Psychosocial Interventions: Evaluation of UNICEF supported projects (1999–2001). UNICEF Indonesia.

Mitchell, J. T. (1983). When disaster strikes . . . The critical incident stress debriefing. *Journal of Emergency Medical Service, 13*(11), 49–52.

Mitchell, J. T., & Everly, G. S. (1996). *Critical incident stress debriefing: An operations manual.* Ellicott City, MD: Chevron.

Mitchell, J. T., & Everly, G. S. (2003). *Critical incident stress management: Group crisis intervention* (3rd ed.). Ellicott City, MD: International Critical Incident Stress Foundation.

Modell, A. H. (1976). "The holding environment" and the therapeutic action of psychoanalysis. *Journal of the American Psychoanalytic Association, 24*, 285–307.

Motta, R. W., Hafeez, S., Sciancalepore, R., & Diaz, A. B. (2001). Discriminant validation of the Modified Secondary Trauma Questionnaire. *Journal of Psychotherapy in Independent Practice, 2*(4), 17–25.

Muñoz, M., Vázquez, J. J., Crespo, M., & Pérez-Santos, E. P. (2004). We were all wounded on March 11th in Madrid: Immediate psychological affects and interventions. *European Psychologist, 9*(4), 278–280.

National Institute for Clinical Excellence. (2005). *Post traumatic stress disorder (PTSD): The management of PTSD in adults and children in primary and secondary care.* London, England: NICE Guidelines.

National Institute for Clinical Excellence. (2005a). *PTSD clinical guidelines.* United Kingdom: NHS.

National Institute for Clinical Excellence. (2005b). *Posttraumatic stress disorder (PTSD): The management of adults and children in primary and secondary care.* United Kingdom: NHS.

National Institute for Health and Care Excellence (2005, March). *Post-traumatic stress disorder (PTSD): The management of PTSD in adults and children in primary and secondary care* (NICE Clinical Guideline 26). London, England: National Institute for Clinical Excellence.

National Institute of Mental Health. (2002). Mental Health and Mass Violence: Evidence-Based Early Psychological Intervention for Victims/Survivors of Mass Violence. A Workshop to Reach Consensus on Best Practices. NIH Publication No. 02–5138, Washington, D.C.: U.S. Government Printing Office.

Nikapota, A. (2006). After the tsunami: A story from Sri Lanka. *International Review of Psychiatry, 18*, 275–279.

Norman, S. B., Stein, M. B., Dimsdale, J. E., & Hoyt, D. B. (2008). Pain in the aftermath of trauma is a risk factor for post-traumatic stress disorder. *Psychology Medicine Journal, 38*, 533–542.

Norris, F. H., Galea, S., Friedman, M. J., & Watson, P. J. (2006). *Methods for disaster mental health research.* New York, NY: Guilford Press.

Nouwen, H. (2010, February). *Nouwen & the Ministry of Presence.* Retrieved from http://missionalchurchnetwork.com/nouwen-the-ministry-of-presence/

Ogden, P., & Minton, K. (2000, January). Sensorimotor psychotherapy: One method for processing traumatic memory. *Traumatology, 4*(3), V1(3), 149–173.

Palm, K. M., Polusny, M. A., & Follette, V. M. (2004). Vicarious traumatization: Potential hazards and interventions for disaster and trauma workers. *Prehospital and Disaster Medicine, 19*(1), 73–78.

Parada, E., & Cervera, M. (Unpublished manuscript, 1997). *Psychological first aid response.* Madrid, Spain: ICAS Spain.

Pearlman, L. A. (1995). Self-care for trauma therapists: Ameliorating vicarious traumatization. In B. H. Stamm (Ed.), *Secondary traumatic stress: Self-care issues for clinicians, researchers, and educators* (pp. 51–64). Lutherville, MD: Sidran Press.

Pearlman, L. A. (1996a). Psychometric review of TSI Belief Scale, Revision L. In B. H. Stamm (Ed.), *Measurement of stress, trauma, and adaptation* (pp. 415–417). Lutherville, MD: Sidran Press.

Pearlman, L. A. (1996b). Psychometric review of TSI Life Event Questionnaire (LEQ). In B. H. Stamm (Ed.), *Measurement of stress, trauma, and adaptation* (pp. 419–430). Lutherville, MD: Sidran Press.

Pearlman, L. A., & Maclan, I. (1995). Vicarious traumatization: An empirical study of the effects of trauma work on trauma therapists. *Professional Psychology: Research and Practice, 26*(6), 558–565.

Pearlmann, L. A., & Saakvitne, K. W. (1995). Trauma and the therapist: Countertransference and vicarious traumatization in psychotherapy with incest survivors. New York, NY: W. W. Norton.

Pellicer, X. (1993). Eye movement desensitization treatment of a child's nightmares: A case report. *Journal of Behavior Therapy and Experimental Psychiatry, 24*, 73–75.

Pennebaker, J. W. (1997). Writing about emotional experiences as a therapeutic process. *Psychological Science,* 8(3), 162–168.

Perkins, B., & Rouanzoin, C. (2002). A critical examination of current views regarding eye movement desensitization and reprocessing (EMDR): Clarifying points of confusion. *Journal of Clinical Psychology, 58,* 77–97.

Puffer, M. K., Greenwald, R., & Elrod, D. E. (1998). A single session EMDR study with twenty traumatized children and adolescents. *Traumatology,* 3(2), Article 6.

Purandare, M., Bhagwagar, H., & Tank, P. (2010, July). *EMDR on children affected by the earthquake.* Paper presented at the 1st EMDR Asia Conference, Bali, Indonesia.

Quinn, G. (2009). Emergency response procedure. In M. Luber (Ed.), *Eye movement and desensitization and reprocessing: Scripted protocols basics and special situations.* New York, NY: Springer.

Radloff, L. S., & Locke, Z. (2000). Center for Epidemiologic Studies Depression Scale (CES-D). In *American Psychiatric Association, task force for the handbook of psychiatric measures* (pp. 523–526). Washington, DC: American Psychiatric Association.

Raphael, B. (1977). Preventive intervention with the recently bereaved. *Archives of General Psychiatry, 34,* 1450–1454.

Reddemann, L. (2009). The inner safe place. In Luber, M. (Ed.), *EMDR Scripted Protocols: Basic and Special Situations* (pp. 71–72). New York, NY: Springer.

Roberts, N. P., Kitchiner, N. J., Kenardy, J., & Bisson, J. I. (2009, March). Systematic review and meta-analysis of multiple-session early interventions following traumatic events. *American Journal of Psychiatry, 166(3),* 293–301. doi: 10.1176/appi.ajp.2008. 08040590

Rudolf, J. (2012, January). *Marines appear to urinate on dead Taliban fighters.* Retrieved from http://www.huffingtonpost.com/2012/01/ll/marines-urinate-corpses-video-afghanistan_n_1200513.html

Russell, A., & O'Connor, M. (2002). Interventions for recovery: The use of EMDR with children in a community-based project. *Association for Child Psychiatry and Psychology, Occasional Paper No. 19,* 43–46.

Russell, M. C. (2006). Treating combat-related stress disorders: Multiple case study utilizing eye movement desensitization and reprocessing (EMDR) with battlefield casualties from the Iraqi war. *Military Psychology, 18,* 1–18.

Russell, M. C. (2008b). Treating traumatic amputation-related phantom limb pain: Case study utilizing eye movement desensitization and reprocessing (EMDR) within the armed services. *Clinical Case Studies, 7,* 136–153.

Russell, M. C. (2008c). War-related medically unexplained symptoms, prevalence and treatment: Utilizing EMDR within the armed services. *Journal of EMDR Practice and Research,* 2(2), 212–225.

Russell, M. C. (2012, January 27). *Preventing military misconduct stress behavior* [Blog]. Retrieved from http://www.huffingtonpost.com/mark-c-russell-phd-abpp/ptsd-veterans_b_l228546.html

Russell, M. C., & Figley, C. F. (2013). *An EMDR practitioners guide to treating traumatic stress disorders in military personnel.* New York, NY: Routledge.

Russell, M. C., & Figley, C. F. (2013). *Treating traumatic stress disorders in military personnel: An EMDR practitioners' guide.* New York, NY: Routledge.

Russell, M. C., Lipke, H. E., & Figley, C. R. (2011). EMDR therapy. In B. A. Moore & W. A. Penk (Eds.), *Handbook for the treatment of PTSD in military personnel.* New York, NY: Guilford Press.

Russell, M. C., Silver, S. M., & Rogers, S. (2007). Responding to an identified need: A joint DoD-DVA training program in EMDR for clinicians providing trauma services. *International Journal of Stress Management,* 14(1), 61–71.

Russell, M. C., Silver, S. M., Rogers, S., & Darnell, J. N. (2007, February). Responding to an identified need: A joint Department of Defense/Department of Veterans Affairs training program in eye movement desensitization and reprocessing (EMDR) for clinicians providing trauma services. International Journal of Stress Management, 14(1), 61–71. doi: 10.1037/1072-5245.14.1.61.

Samec, J. (2001). The use of EMDR safe place exercise in group therapy with traumatized adolescent refugees [Special edition]. *The EMDRIA Newsletter*. 32–34

Scheck, M. M., Schaeffer, J. A., & Gillette, C. S. (1998). Brief psychological intervention with traumatized young women: The efficacy of eye movement desensitization and reprocessing. *Journal of Traumatic Stress, 11*, 25–44.

Schwartz, A. C., Bradley, R., Penza, K. M., Sexton, M., Jay, D., Haggard, P. J., . . . Ressler, K. J. (2006). Pain medicine use among patients with posttraumatic stress disorder. *Psychosomatics, 47*, 136–142.

Shacham, Y. (2009, January). Challenges in extending help cross culturally [Unpublished PowerPoint slides]. Paper presented at the International Conference on Crisis as an Opportunity: Organizational and Professional Responses to Disaster, Ben-Gurion University of the Negev, Beersheva, Israel.

Shalev, A. Y., Ankri, Y., Israeli-Shalev, Y., Peleg, T., Adessky, R., & Freedman, S. (2012). Prevention of posttraumatic stress disorder by early treatment: Results from the Jerusalem Trauma Outreach and Prevention study. *Archives for General Psychiatry, 69*(2), 166–176.

Shani, Z. (2006, July). *Group EMDR with school children following a traumatic event*. Invited presentation at EMDR-Israel HAP conference, Netanya, Israel.

Shapiro, F. (2006). *EMDR: New notes on adaptive information processing with case formulation principles, forms, scripts and worksheets*. Watsonville, CA: EMDR Institute.

Shapiro, E. (2009). EMDR treatment of recent trauma events. *Journal of EMDR Practice and Research, 3*(3), 141–151.

Shapiro, E., & Laub, B., (2008a). Early EMDR intervention (EEI): Summary, a theoretical model, and the recent traumatic episode protocol (R-TEP). *Journal of EMDR Practice and Research, 2*(2), 79–96.

Shapiro, E., & Laub, B., (2008b, May). *Unfinished-traumatic episode protocol (U-TEP) A new protocol for early EMDR interventions*. Paper presented at the EMDR Europe Annual Conference, London, England.

Shapiro, E., & Laub, B. (2009). The recent traumatic episode protocol (R-TEP): An integrative protocol for early EMDR intervention (EEI). In M. Luber (Ed.), *Eye movement and desensitization and reprocessing: Scripted protocols basics and special situations* (pp. 251–270). New York, NY: Springer.

Shapiro, F. (1989). Efficacy of eye movement desensitization procedure in the treatment of traumatic memory. *Journal of Traumatic Stress, 2*(2), 199–223.

Shapiro, F. (1989). Eye movement desensitization. A new treatment for posttraumatic stress disorder. *Journal of Behavior Therapy and Experimental Psychiatry, 20*, 211–217.

Shapiro, F. (1991). Eye movement desensitization and reprocessing procedure: From EMD to EMDR: A new treatment model for anxiety and related traumata. *Behavior Therapist, 14*, 133–135.

Shapiro, F. (1995). *Eye movement desensitization and reprocessing: Basic principles, protocols, and procedures* (1st ed.). New York, NY: Guilford Press.

Shapiro, F. (2001). *Eye movement desensitization and reprocessing: basic principles, protocols, and procedures* (2nd ed.). New York, NY: Guilford Press.

Shapiro, F. [scripted by M. Luber].(2009). Recent traumatic events protocol. In Luber, M. (Ed.), *EMDR scripted protocols: Basic and special situations* (pp. 143–154). New York, NY: Springer.

Shapiro, F. (2006). *New notes on adaptive information processing with case formulation principles, forms, scripts, and worksheets*. Watsonville, CA: EMDR Institute.

Silver, S. M., Rogers, S., Knipe, J., & Colelli, G. (2005). EMDR therapy following the 9/11 terrorist attacks: A community-based intervention project in New York City. *International Journal of Stress Management, 12*, 29–42.

Silver, S. M., Rogers, S., & Russell, M. (2008). Eye movement desensitization and reprocessing (EMDR) in the treatment of war veterans. *Journal of Clinical Psychology: In session, 64*(8), 947–957.

Skovholt, T. M. (2001). *The resilient practitioner: Burnout prevention and self-care strategies for counsellors, therapists, teachers, and health professionals*. Boston, MA: Allyn & Bacon.

Soberman, G. B., Greenwald, R., & Rule, D. L. (2002). A controlled study of eye movement desensitization and reprocessing (EMDR) for boys with conduct problems. *Journal of Aggression, Maltreatment, and Trauma, 6*, 217–236.

Solomon, R. (2008). Critical incident interventions. *Journal of EMDR Practice and Research, 2*, 160–165.

Solomon, R. M. (1988, October). Post-shooting trauma, *Police Chief*, pp. 40–44.

Solomon, R. M., & Horn, J. M. (1986). Post-shooting traumatic. In J. Reese & H. Goldstein (Eds.), *Law enforcement* (pp. 383–393). Washington, DC: United States Government Printing Office.

Spielberger, C. D., Gorssuch, R. L., Lushene, P. R., Vagg, P. R., & Jacobs, G. A. (1983). *Manual for the State-Trait Anxiety Inventory*. Palo Alto, CA: Consulting Psychologists Press.

Stamm, B. H. (2010). *The Concise ProQOL manual* (2nd ed.). Pocatello, ID: ProQOL.org

Stewart, K., & Bramson, T. (2000). Incorporating EMDR in residential treatment. *Residential Treatment for Children & Youth, 17*, 83–90.

Strupp, H. H., & Binder, J. L. (1984). *Psychotherapy in a new key: A guide to time-limited dynamic psychotherapy*. New York, NY: Basic Books.

Tank, P. (2011). *A presentation on EMDR*. Delhi, India: ANCIPS, EMDR.

Taylor, R. (2002). Family unification with reactive attachment disorder: A brief treatment. *Contemporary Family Therapy: An International Journal, 24*, 475–481.

Tedeschi, R., & Calhoun, L. (1995). *Trauma and transformation: Growing in the aftermath of suffering*. Thousand Oaks, CA: Sage.

Tedeschi, R., & Calhoun, L. (2004). Posttraumatic growth: Conceptual foundations and evidence, *Psychological Inquiry, 15(l)*, 1–18.

Tinker, R. H., & Wilson, S. A. (1999). *Through the eyes of a child: EMDR with children*. New York, NY: W. W. Norton.

Turkish Psychological Association. (1999). *Annual bulletin*. Ankara: Author.

U.S. Department of Veterans Affairs & US Department of Defense. (2004). *VA/DoD clinical practice guideline for the management of post-traumatic stress*. Washington, D.C.

Ullmann, E., & Hilweg, W. (2000). *Infancia y Trauma, separación, abuso y guerra*. Auryn colección. Brand. Madrid. (German Original version, 1997).

Van Peski, C. (2006, January). *CSPC crisis intervention training Colombo, Sri Lanka*. Unpublished manuscript, Community Stress Prevention Center, Kiryat Shmona, Israel.

Van Rooyen, M., & Leaning, J. (2005). After the tsunami: Facing the public health challenges. *New England Journal of Medicine, 352*, 435–438.

Weathers, F., Litz, B., Herman, D., Huska, J., & Keane, T. (1993). *The PTSD Checklist (PCL): Reliability, validity, and diagnostic utility*. Paper presented at the annual meeting of the International Society for Traumatic Stress studies, San Antonio, TX.

Weiss, D. S., & Marmar, C. R. (1996). The Impact of Event Scale—Revised. In J. Wilson & T. M. Keane (Eds.), *Assessing psychological trauma and PTSD* (1st ed., pp. 399–411). New York, NY: Guilford Press.

Wesson, M., & Gould, M. (2009). Intervening early with EMDR on military operations. *Journal of EMDR Practice and Research*, 3(2), 91–97.

White, M., & Epston, D. (1990). *Narrative means to therapeutic ends*. New York: Norton.

Wilson, S., Tinker, R., Hofmann, A., Becker, L., & Marshall, S. (2000). *A field study of EMDR with Kosovar-Albanian refugee children using a group treatment protocol*. Paper presented at the annual meeting of the International Society for the Study of Traumatic Stress, San Antonio, TX.

World Health Organization Quality of Life. (1995). Position paper from the World Health Organization. *Social Science and Medicine, 41*(10), 1403–1409.

Zaghrout-Hodali, M., Alissa, F., & Dodgson, P. (2008). Building resilience and dismantling fear: EMDR group protocol with children in an area of ongoing trauma. *Journal of EMDR Practice and Research, 2, 106.*

Zeidner, M., & Hadar, D. (2012, July). Psychoactualia, secondary traumatization among trauma therapists [Hebrew]. *Quarterly of the Israeli Psychological Association*, 42–52.

Additional Readings

Alayarian, A. (2007). Trauma, resilience and creativity: Examining our therapeutic approach in working with refugees. *European Journal of Psychotherapy, Counselling & Health, 9*(3), 313–324.

Altan Aytun, O., Ozcan, G., Ciftci, A., Konuk, E., Yuksek, H., Karakus, D., . . . Vatan Ozcelik, D. (2010, June). The effects of early EMDR interventions (EMD and R-TEP) on the victims of a terrorist bombing in Istanbul. In *Treatment of children/acute stress.* Symposium conducted at the annual meeting of the EMDR Europe Association, Hamburg, Germany.

American Psychological Association. (2003). The road to resilience. Retrieved from http://www.apa.Org/helpcenter/road-resilience.aspx#

Ayalon, O., Lahad, M., & Cohen, A. (1999). *Community stress prevention* (Vols. 3, 4). Kiryat Shmona, Israel: The Community Stress Prevention Center, Jerusalem Ministry of Education.

Bados, A., Toribio, L., & García-Grau, E. (2008). Traumatic events and tonic immobility. *The Spanish Journal of Psychology, 11*(2), 516–521.

Blore, D., & Holmshaw, M. (2009). EMDR blind to therapist protocol. In M. Luber (Ed.), *Eye movement desensitization and reprocessing (EMDR) scripted protocols: Basic and special situations* (pp. 233–240). New York, NY: Springer.

Bremner, J. D. (2005). *Does stress damage the brain? Understanding trauma-related disorders from a mind-body perspective.* New York, NY: W. W. Norton.

Breslau, N., Chilcoat, H. D., Kessler, R. C., & Davis, G. C. (1999). Previous exposure to trauma and PTSD effects of subsequent trauma: Results from the Detroit area survey of trauma. *American Journal of Psychiatry, 156*(6), 902–907.

Brill, N. Q., & Beebe, G. W. (1952). Psychoneurosis: Military application of a follow-up study. *U.S. Armed Forces Medicine Journal, 3*, 15–33.

Brunet, A., Weiss, D. S., Metzler, T. J., Best, S. R., Neylan, T. C., Rogers, C., . . . Marmar, C. R. (2001). The Peritraumatic Distress Inventory: A proposed measure of PTSD criterion A2. *American Journal of Psychiatry, 158*, 1480–1485.

Brymer, J., Layne, P., Ruzek, S., & Vernberg, W. (2006). *Psychological first aid (PFA).* Los Angeles, CA: National Child Traumatic Stress Network and National Center for PTSD.

Bui, E., Brunet, A., Allenou, C., Camassel, C., Raynaud, J. P., Claudet, I., . . . Birmes, P. (2010). Peritraumatic reactions and posttraumatic stress symptoms in school-aged children victims of road traffic accident. *General Hospital Psychiatry, 32*, 330–333.

Carlson, J. G., Chemtob, C. M., Rusnack, K., Hedlund, N. L., & Muraoka, M. Y. (1998). Eye movement desensitization and reprocessing for combat-related posttraumatic stress disorder. *Journal of Traumatic Stress, 11*, 3–24.

Carmelo, V., Gonzalo, H., & Perez-Sales, P. (2008). Chronic thought suppression and posttraumatic symptoms: Data from the Madrid March 11, 2004 terrorist attack. *Journal of Anxiety Disorders, 22*, 1326–1336.

Cervera, M. (2006). La técnica EMDR en la práctica Terapéutica. La empresa privada en la intervención psicológica en desastres: ICAS. In R. Ramos (Ed.), *Psicología Aplicada a Crisis, Desastres y Catástrofes.* Melilla, Spain: UNED Centro Asociado.

Cervera, M. (2012). La intervencion en situatciones de crisis en las empresas y los primeros auxilios psicólogos. In L. N. Martin & A. S. Sordo (Eds.), *Tratando Situaciones de Emergencia* (pp. 195–210). Madrid, Spain: Pirámide.

Chossegros, L., Hours, M., Charnay, P., Bernard, M., Fort, E., Boisson, D., . . . Laumon, B. (2011). Predictive factors of chronic post-traumatic stress disorder 6 months after a road accident. *Accident Analysis and Prevention, 43*, 471–477.

Creamer, M., Bell, R., & Failla, S. (2003). Psychometric properties of the Impact of Event Scale-Revised. *Behaviour Research and Therapy, 41*, 1489–1496.

Department of the Army. (2009). *Combat and operational stress control manual for leaders and soldiers: Field Manual No. 6-22-5*. Washington, DC: Headquarters, Department of the Army.

Department of Veteran's Affairs & Department of Defense. (2004). *VA/DoD clinical practice guideline for the management of post-traumatic stress* (Office of Quality and Performance Publication 10Q-CPG/PTSD-04). Washington, DC: Veterans Health Administration, Department of Veterans Affairs and Health Affairs, Department of Defense.

Dyregov, A., & Mitchell, J. (1992). Work with traumatized children; Psychological effects and working strategies. *Journal of Traumatic Stress, 5*(1), 5–17.

Fernández-Liria, A., & Rodríguez-Vega, B. (2002). *Intervención en crisis*. Madrid, Spain: Síntesis.

Figley, C. R., & Nash, W. P. (2007). *Combat stress injury: Theory, research, and management*. New York, NY: Routledge.

Finely, E. P., Baker, M., Pugh, M. J., & Peterson, A. (2010). Intimate partner violence committed by returning veterans with post-traumatic stress disorder. *Journal of Family Violence, 25*, 737–743.

Foa, E. B., Keane, T. M., & Friedman, M. J. (Eds.). (2000). *Effective treatments for PTSD: Practice guidelines from the International Society for Traumatic Stress Studies*. New York, NY: Guilford Press.

Galliano, S. (2002). Debriefing reconsidered. *Counseling and Psychotherapy Journal, 3*(2), 20–21.

Gendlin, E. (2002). *Focusing, proceso y técnica de enfoque corporal*. Bilbao, Spain: Mensajero.

Gentry, J. (1999). *Compassion satisfaction manual* (p. 25). Toronto, Canada: Psych Ink Resources.

Gibson, L. E. (2004). *Acute stress disorder: A brief description*. A National Center for PTSD Fact Sheet (www.ncptsd.org).

Gilbar, O., Plivazky, N., & Gil, S. (2010). Counterfactual thinking, coping strategies, and coping resources as predictors of PTSD diagnosed in physically injured victims of terror attacks. *Journal of Loss and Trauma, 15*, 304–324.

Gordon, R. (2007). Thirty years of trauma work: Clarifying and broadening the consequences of trauma. *Psychotherapy in Australia, 13*(3), 12–19.

Grossman, D. (1996). *On killing: The psychological cost of learning to kill in war and society*. Toronto, ON: Little, Brown.

Guenthner, D. H. (2012). Emergency and crisis management: Critical incident stress management for first responders and business organizations. *Journal of Business Continuing Emergency Plan, 5*(4), 298–315.

Horowitz, M. J. (1976). *Stress response syndromes*. New York, NY: Jason Aronson.

Horowitz, M. J. (1999). Signs and symptoms of posttraumatic stress disorder. In M. J. Horowitz (Ed.), *Essential papers on posttraumatic stress disorder* (pp. 1–17). New York, NY: New York University Press.

Institute of Medicine. (2008). *Gulf War and health: Volume 6. Physiologic, psychologic and psychosocial effects of deployment-related stress*. Washington, DC: National Academies Press.

International Association of Firefighters. (2001). *Guide to developing fire service labor/ employee assistance & critical incident stress management programs*. Retrieved from http://www.iaff.org/hs/LODD_Manual/Resources/IAFF%20Developing%20Fire%20Service%20Labor-Employee%20Assistance%20and%20CISM%20Programs.pdf

Kimbrel, S., Meyer, K., Knight, Z., & Gulliver. (2011). A revised measure of occupational stress for firefighters: Psychometric properties and relationship to posttraumatic stress disorder, depression, and substance abuse. *Psychological Services*, 8(4), 294–306.

Knipe, J., Hartung, J., Konuk, E., Colelli, G., Keller, M., & Rogers, S. (2003, September). *EMDR Humanitarian Assistance Programs: Outcome research, models of training, and service delivery in New York, Latin America, Turkey and Indonesia*. Symposium conducted at the annual meeting of the EMDR at the annual meeting of the EMDR Europe Association, Istanbul, Turkey.

Konuk, E. (2002). *The August and November 1999 Turkish earthquakes: An EMDR HAP progress report*. The EMDR Practitioner. Retrieved from http://www.emdrpractitioner.net/

Korn, D. L., Weir, J., & Rozelle, D. (2004). *Looking beyond the data: Clinical lessons learned from an EMDR treatment outcome study*. Paper presented at the EMDR International Association Conference, Montreal, Canada.

Kutz, I., Resnik, V., & Dekel, R. (2008). The effect of single-session modified EMDR on acute stress syndromes. *Journal of EMDR Practice and Research*, 2(3), 190–200.

Lazarus, A. (1989). *The practice of multimodal therapy*. New York, NY: McGraw-Hill.

Leach, J. (2004). Why people "freeze" in an emergency. Temporal and cognitive constraint on survival response. *Aviation, Space, and Environmental Medicine*, 75, 539–542.

Levine, P. (2008). *Healing trauma: A pioneering program for restoring the wisdom of your body*. Berkeley, CA: North Atlantic Books.

Shapiro, F. [scripted by M. Luber]. (2009). Recent traumatic events protocol. In Luber, M. (Ed.), *EMDR scripted protocols: Basic and special situations* (pp. 143–154). New York, NY: Springer.

Marks, I. M. (1987). *Fears, phobias and rituals: Panic, anxiety and their disorders*. Oxford, England: Oxford University Press. (Spanish translation: *Miedos, fobias y rituals 1: Los mecanismos de la ansiedad*. Barcelona: Martínez Roca, 1991.)

Marshall, G. N., Davis, L. M., & Sherbourne, C. D. (2000). *A review of the scientific literature as it pertains to Gulf War illnesses: Volume 4 stress*. Prepared for the Office of the Secretary of Defense. National Defense Research Institute, RAND, Santa Monica, CA.

McNally, R. J., Bryant, R. A., & Ehlers, A. (2003). Does early psychological intervention promote recovery from posttraumatic stress? *Psychological Science in the Public Interest*, 4(2), 45–79.

Meyer, E. C., Zimering, R., Daly, E., Knight, J., Kamholz, B. W., & Gulliver, S. (2012). Predictors of posttraumatic stress disorder and other psychological symptoms in trauma-exposed firefighters. *Psychological Services*, 9(1), 1–15.

Mitchell, J. T., & Everly, G. S. (2001). Critical incident stress management and critical incident stress debriefing: Evolution, effects and outcomes. In B. Raphael & J. Wilson (Eds.), *Psychological debriefing: Theory, practice and evidence*. Cambridge, UK: Cambridge University Press.

Murphy, S. A., Bond, G. E., Beaton, R. D., Murphy, J., & Clark, L. C. (2002). Lifestyle practices and occupational stressors as predictors of health outcomes in urban firefighters. *International Journal of Stress Management*, 9(4), 311–327.

Neria, Y., DiGrande, L., & Adams, B. G. (2011). Posttraumatic stress disorder following the September 11, 2001, terrorist attacks: A review of the literature among highly exposed populations. *American Psychologist*, 66(6), 429–446.

Ogden, P., Minton, K., & Pain, C. (2006). *Trauma and the body: A sensorimotor approach to psychotherapy*. New York, NY: W. W. Norton.

Rothschild, B. (2006). *Help for the helper: Self-care strategies for managing burnout and stress*. New York, NY: W. W. Norton.

Russell, M. C. (2008a). Scientific resistance to research, training, and utilization of EMDR therapy in treating post-war disorders. *Social Science and Medicine, 67*(11), 1737–1746.

Russell, M. C., & Friedberg, F. (2009). Training, treatment access and research on trauma intervention in the armed services. *Journal of EMDR Practice and Research*, 3, 24–31.

Seyle, H., & Fortier, C. (1950). Adaptive reaction to stress. *Psychosomatic Medicine 12(3)*, 149–157.

Shapiro, E. (2007). 4 Elements exercise. *Journal of EMDR Practice and Research*, 2, 113–115.

Shapiro, E. (2012). EMDR and early psychological intervention following trauma. *European Journal of Applied Psychology (ERAP)*, V. 62(4), 241–251.

Shapiro, F. (1993). Eye movement desensitization and reprocessing (EMDR). *Journal of Traumatic Stress*, 6, 417–421.

Shapiro, F. (1999). Eye movement desensitization and reprocessing (EMDR) and the anxiety disorders: Clinical and research implications of an integrated psychotherapy treatment. *Journal of Anxiety Disorders, 13*(1–2, Excerpt), 35–67.

Shapiro, F. (2004). *Military and post-disaster field manual*. Hamden, CT: EMDR Humanitarian Assistance Program.

Shapiro, F. (In press). Protocol for recent traumatic events. In M. Luber (Ed.), *Implementing EMDR early mental health interventions for man-made and natural disasters: Models, scripted protocols and summary sheets*. New York, NY: Springer.

Silver, S., & Rogers, S. (2001). *Light in the heart of darkness: EMDR and the treatment of war and terrorism survivors*. New York, NY: W. W. Norton.

Slonim, D. (2010, July). *Post traumatic stress disorder*. Paper presented at the NATO Science for Peace conference, Istanbul, Turkey.

Sosa, C. D., & Capafons, J. (2005). *Estrés Postraumático*. Madrid, Spain: Síntesis.

Stapert, M., & Verliefde, E. (2008). *Focusing with children. The art of communicating with children at school and at home*. United Kingdom: PCCS Books. (Spanish versión 2011.)

Ullmann, E., & Hilweg, W. (2000). *Infancia y Trauma, separación, abuso y guerra*. Auryn colección. Madrid: Brand. (German Original version, 1997.) Wittman, L., Zehnder, D., Schredl, M., Jenni, O. G., & Landolt, M. A. (2010). Posttraumatic nightmares and psychopathology in children after a road traffic accidents. *Journal of Traumatic Stress*, 23(2), 232–239.

Yehuda, R. (1999). *Risk factors for posttraumatic stress disorder*. Washington, DC: American Psychiatric Association. Yehuda, R. (2001). Biology of post traumatic stress disorder. *Psychiatric Clinics of North America, 62*(Suppl. 17), 41–46.

Zayfer, C., & Becker, C. B. (2007). *Cognitive—Behavioral therapy for PTSD*. New York, NY: Guilford Press. (Spanish versión, 2008. México: El Manual Moderno.)

www.ingramcontent.com/pod-product-compliance
Ingram Content Group UK Ltd.
Pitfield, Milton Keynes, MK11 3LW, UK
UKHW050459150426
5217IPUK00025B/1751